STO

A WOMAN TALKS WITH HER DOCTOR

A Comprehensive Guide to Women's Health Care

A WOMAN TALKS WITH HER DOCTOR

A Comprehensive
Guide to
Women's Health Care

CHARLES E. FLOWERS, JR., M.D.
and MAXINE ABRAMS

WILLIAM MORROW AND COMPANY, INC.
NEW YORK   1979

Library of Congress Cataloging in Publication Data

Flowers, Charles E.
　　A woman talks with her doctor.

　　Includes index.
　　1. Gynecology—Popular works.　2. Obstetrics—
Popular works.　I. Abrams, Maxine, joint author.
II. Title.
RG121.F56　　　618　　　　79-9766
ISBN　0-688-03458-6

BOOK DESIGN　　CARL WEISS

Printed in the United States of America.

First Edition

1　2　3　4　5　6　7　8　9　10

To

JUANZETTA

AND SIDNEY

ACKNOWLEDGMENTS

The authors wish to thank:

Susan Ann Protter for initiating the collaboration which made this book possible;

Robert Bender for his thoughtful editorial guidance;

Juanzetta Flowers for her help with the chapter on sexuality;

Mary Barnes for her devotion to this project and long hours of secretarial service;

Dr. William Huggins for his careful review of the manuscript;

Jeanne Dunphey for the preparation of the illustrations;

Edmond J. Murray for the jacket photograph.

CONTENTS

A WOMAN TALKS WITH HER DOCTOR

A Comprehensive Guide to Women's Health Care

1

GETTING ACQUAINTED

Dr. Flowers, could I ask you first why a man becomes a gynecologist?

I can only tell you that *I* became a gynecologist-obstetrician because I felt that I had a lot of empathy with women. I gradually began to realize this while I was in college.

One day, for instance, I had a swimming date with a girl who began to menstruate heavily through her bathing suit. She was very upset, but I found that I wasn't embarrassed at all. I gave her my handkerchief and told her, "Don't worry about it. Menstruation is perfectly normal."

Possibly my attitude came from being raised near my grandfather's farm, where I was around animals a great deal. I considered the reproductive process natural and very important.

Later, as I completed my medical education, I began to realize that obstetrics and gynecology combined some of the most important and pleasant aspects of the practice of medicine. I was attracted by the combination of internal medicine, surgery, psychiatry and endocrinology.

But don't you think that a woman gynecologist has a communication edge over a man?

I know the ones that I work with do. They are intelligent and they like women, and I think the male gynecologists learn a great deal from them. Women physicians are better able to communicate with women patients simply because they share similar experiences. After all, a male gynecologist-obstetrician can never really know what it is like to menstruate, to experience a female orgasm or to birth a baby.

I also believe that a woman gynecologist, or a sensitive nurse practitioner, can take a sexual and marital history much better than the average male physician. There are, of course, some men who can make women feel very comfortable, but I believe a woman physician does have a communication edge—as long as she uses it properly, with empathy and understanding.

That being the case, why should a woman go to a male gynecologist?

There is more to gynecology and obstetrics than sexual history taking, and there are many fine physicians of both sexes. The chemistry inherent in a good doctor-patient relationship is more a matter of personality, and a woman should choose the physician with whom she feels most comfortable and in whom she has the most confidence.

The choosing of a doctor often comes down to a matter of personal preference. As in everything else, there are differences of opinion— just as there are differences in the various approaches physicians take with their patients. So I think we should look for a "fit" in a physician, just as we look for a fit in everything else in our lives.

What's the best way to find a good doctor?

There are many fine doctors, and there is nothing at all wrong with shopping around. One good starting point might be a recommendation from another doctor or from a friend or neighbor. A woman can also call the most reputable medical center in her area and request assistance. Ultimately, however, she is going to have to judge the doctor for herself. So she should ask herself, Is this physician genuinely interested in my problem? Does he take the time to get to know and understand me? Does he make it easy for me to confide in him? Will he honor my confidences and respect my intelligence and my wishes?

If a doctor doesn't do all this, the woman should keep looking until she finds one who does. She is under no obligation to the doctor, but it is courteous to break any appointment she may have made.

And another thing. Just because a woman has been with a doctor for many years doesn't mean she must stay with him forever. Women have the darnedest reasons for remaining with a physician, even when he is getting too old. They don't want to hurt his feelings. But there comes a time when a woman must say to herself, "My body is more important than my loyalty to this doctor."

But the very nature of the doctor-patient relationship seems so intimidating, so unequal. Obviously the physician has more information.

That is true, but the doctor's training and education do not give him license to make all the decisions or to treat the patient as an inferior being. If a woman feels this is happening in her relationship with her physician, it is her responsibility to speak up.

This, in fact, is exactly what has been happening in recent years. Women have been taking more responsibility for their own health and the doctor-patient relationship has undergone a drastic revision. Patients now realize that physicians have no magic wands, and we are seeing growing numbers of intelligent women who say to themselves,

"I'm just as smart as this doctor, except he had a different type of education. I expect us to work together on my health problems. I would like to have him as my coach, so to speak, but I am the one in charge of me."

Often the intimidation is quite subtle. An unspoken attitude on the part of many doctors seems to imply, How dare you not do what I say or question my judgment?

It is true there are some doctors in all specialties who project themselves as authoritative father figures. They remain aloof, looking down on the patient, and their attitude is not as thoughtful, kind, and caring as it should be.

If a woman is pregnant, this type of doctor will decide what she must eat, when she may have sexual relations and when she may travel. He may even enjoy having such complete control over many of her important and intimate activities. Unfortunately he never says, "Let's talk about some of your thoughts and fears."

Oppressive as this may sound, there are some women who actually like this sort of doctor. They want the doctor to do it all, and they leave his office very comfortable that he has "laid hands" on them and has given them a clean bill of health.

These women need to be honest with themselves. They must be made to understand they are paying a price for this pseudosecurity. They are relinquishing control over many of the important decisions involving their own body.

What other mistakes do women make in dealing with doctors?

Probably the most common mistake is not being willing to make the effort to find a caring, competent physician. And the second mistake is not communicating with him fully once you have found him.

The human body is the most complex and the most beautifully programmed machine on earth, and there are thousands of things that can go wrong or that can worry you. There is no way the doctor can know all the potential problems without your telling him. If you took your car to a mechanic you would certainly describe its symptoms. And if he didn't fix it properly, you'd bring it back.

So just remember, the doctor is not omniscient. He has no way of knowing what your emotions are or how your body feels. If you want him to look for something in particular, for goodness' sake, tell him. It's your responsibility.

Still another common mistake is failure to follow instructions. If you go to a doctor you have confidence in, you should do what he tells you. Let's say you have vaginitis and your doctor tells you not to wear underclothes around the house. He has a very good reason for issuing these instructions. Your vaginitis will become worse if you keep your bottom wrapped up all the time, and the bacteria and yeast have a warm, moist environment in which to grow. Of course, it is important for your physician to explain your illness and its treatment clearly and completely. You need this information to participate more intelligently in your care.

What are the most common mistakes doctors make in dealing with patients?

Physicians often do not set the proper environment or make certain the patient is comfortable and relaxed so they can develop the necessary dialogue. For instance, an amazing number of women tell me that no physician has ever taken even a brief sexual history from them. I realize it is possible that a doctor may have taken such a history in a casual sort of way so that the patient was unaware, but I am afraid that many doctors do not set the proper environment for this type of discussion. They themselves are not relaxed with the subject, and they feel threatened when they discuss a patient's sexuality.

Now I'm not saying I always do a good job of putting the patient at ease. Maybe one day I am particularly busy, or I have a problem on my mind. Maybe I forget one important question. Then it's up to the patient to help me discover her problem, to tell me if I miss something. Or if I do not offer a clear explanation that the patient can understand, then it's up to her to reopen the discussion and indicate its importance to her.

Here again, it's a matter of good, clear communication, and I repeatedly caution medical students to make certain they have been properly understood in their conversations with patients. Even so, there can be occasional misunderstanding on both sides.

What kind of misunderstanding?

I have had women actually become insulted that I would ask intimate questions, and I have been accused of being a "dirty old man" because I have inquired about the frequency of intercourse, the frequency of orgasmic response and the adequacy of lubrication. Some patients have blushed or turned their head away and said, "I've never had a doctor ask me these questions before. I really don't like to answer them."

Of course, I explain that these are important questions, and if there are any problems I may be able to help. Nevertheless, it is a woman's privilege not to answer them if they are offensive to her.

There can also be misunderstandings when there are marital problems. One patient thought I was trying to get information that would be of assistance to her husband in divorce proceedings.

Still another kind of misinterpretation can occur when patients come to a gynecologist with complex medical problems. I remember one patient who had both gall-bladder disease and pelvic infection. The gall bladder was on her mind, and the infection was on my mind. When we began to discuss the situation, it became clear that her answers and remarks were totally inappropriate, and it was necessary to define the problems we were discussing in order to find out how I could be of assistance to her.

What other problems can a woman bring to an obstetrician-gynecologist? What are the limits of his expertise?

The well-trained obstetrician-gynecologist is a specialist in pregnancy and childbirth as well as in diseases of the female pelvis and reproductive organs. These diseases may range from vaginal infections to fibroid tumors to cancer. The majority of gynecologists are also competent in managing urinary-tract infections, certain forms of urinary incontinence (where a woman loses urine when she coughs or sneezes), and other difficulties associated with the urinary process. A gynecologist can also treat minor rectal problems, including hemorrhoids.

The obstetrician-gynecologist is also trained to provide pre-conception counseling and to assist with fertility problems. One of his most important responsibilities is to manage the patient through a safe and healthy pregnancy, labor, and delivery.

Do obstetrician-gynecologists specialize in certain areas?

Indeed they do, and this trend is increasing. There are now gynecologic subspecialists in maternal and fetal medicine, endocrinology and infertility, and cancer. These obstetrician-gynecologists have completed the regular forty-eight-month postgraduate training following their M.D. degree and have taken two or more additional years in a special fellowship in their field of interest. There is no question they have special competence in their particular division of obstetrics and gynecology.

The physicians in maternal and fetal medicine are particularly competent to treat women who have high-risk problems of pregnancy, such as diabetes, hypertension, the Rh problem, or heart, kidney, or liver disease.

The physician who has special training in endocrinology and infertility is particularly competent to diagnose hormonal disorders and to treat women who have problems conceiving.

The gynecologic oncologist is skilled in the surgical treatment of cancer of the pelvis. The well-trained gynecologic oncologist collaborates with a team including other surgical specialists, radiation therapists, and chemotherapists so that the treatment is directed to the patient's specific needs.

Is it wise for a woman to use her gynecologist as her family doctor?

Studies have shown that 60 percent of all women in this country do consider their gynecologist-obstetrician their primary physician. This is an excellent trend in that it reduces the number of physicians a woman must have in order to meet most of her health-care needs. If the obstetrician-gynecologist is competent in the complex problems of his specialty, it is obvious he can treat many of the nuisance illnesses which occur from time to time.

Moreover, the doctor and patient have probably established a good rapport. They probably communicate well, and it is often simple for him to provide her total care. When necessary, he can refer her to other specialists for treatment outside his realm of expertise or interest.

Whether a woman *wishes* to use her obstetrician-gynecologist as her primary physician will depend upon her personality, how she feels about her doctor and his availability.

How can a woman judge her doctor's credentials?

There are varying degrees of intelligence and competence among physicians, just as there are among lawyers, educators, engineers, and automobile mechanics. Moreover, great brilliance is not always necessary. What is required is a thoughtful, competent physician who works well with a particular patient and who turns to other competent, caring specialists as they are needed. Such a team will accomplish much more in delivery of effective obstetric and gynecologic care than a brilliant physician who is not attuned to the patient's needs or is uninterested in her minor complaints.

Neither is it always possible to judge a doctor's competence by the college, university, or even medical school he attended. However, a good rule of thumb is this: if an obstetrician-gynecologist took his residency in an outstanding medical center, he will probably be an excellent obstetrician-gynecologist. Even then, however, his personality and approach might not appeal to an individual patient.

Another way to evaluate the excellence of an obstetrician-gynecologist is by the hospital in which he has privileges. A well-trained obstetrician-gynecologist will be on the staff of an institution which is well regarded in the community. Ideally, he should also be board-certified in his specialty. One must always be cautious, however, about selecting a physician in small, private, and proprietary hospitals.

How can a woman tell whether her doctor is staying abreast of recent medical advances?

This is sometimes difficult for a lay person to do, but if a woman is going to a physician who works in a medical center or medical-school hospital, she can be reasonably sure her physician's information is up to date. These hospitals are constantly having conferences on the latest developments, and, even more important, they have regular peer reviews, which are general discussions and examination of complications that have occurred in that hospital. Unfortunately, in many hospitals in our country, errors and mistakes are committed and never discussed, and there is no real peer pressure to develop and maintain excellence.

Of course, a physician who is not associated with a large medical center or university hospital can also remain current if he reads the medical literature and attends appropriate postgraduate programs and conferences in his own hospital. Fortunately the American College of Obstetricians and Gynecologists and the American College of Family Practice are requiring attendance at postgraduate programs and recertification, for which a doctor must take an exam ten years after obtaining his degree.

Suppose a woman is under treatment by a gynecologist and she is not satisfied with her progress?

Then she should ask for a special appointment in order to have a frank discussion with her physician. She should state quite candidly, "I'm not satisfied with how I'm getting along, and I really don't understand my illness and what we're doing about it. I would like to arrange another appointment as soon as possible so we can discuss my problems further while they're still fresh in your mind."

During this conference, the woman should ask the doctor to illustrate her problem with a drawing. Then if she still does not understand her illness or continues to be dissatisfied with her treatment or her progress, it is proper for her to ask for a consultation with another specialist.

What if a woman has difficulty verbalizing her concerns? Some women are out the door before they have asked all their questions.

One way to be certain that the doctor will answer all your questions is to put them in writing before the visit. Make a list and take it with you. This list will help you remember all your questions and probably allow you to feel more relaxed during your visit.

Many women feel particularly pressured when they are facing an important decision—for instance, whether or not to have an operation.

It is *extremely* important that women not allow themselves to be rushed when it comes to making such decisions. There are very few emergencies that can't wait for a thoughtful decision by the patient and her family, if their opinion is important.

Many women tell me about surgery which they consider to have been unnecessary, and I ask them, "Why did you allow it?" They say, "My doctor put me in the hospital that very day, and I had my womb out before I knew what was happening." But all they had to say was, "Wait a minute. I'm not ready to have this done. I want to think about it. This is a serious decision for me. I would like to talk this over with my husband or lover or friends or family. Would it be all right if they called you to talk to you about this?"

Women simply have to find the confidence to speak out under these circumstances even if they must resort to memorization of a simple speech. If they are timid, they should promise themselves *before* the visit that they will not make any decisions they have not had a chance to think over.

If I see that a patient is hesitant about my advice, I encourage her to take her time and I suggest that she seek another opinion—or two or three. It's worth the money to have peace of mind, and a woman should never be afraid of hurting the doctor's feelings. A competent physician welcomes a consultation. If a doctor becomes angry or threatened when he is asked for a consultation, then the patient really *needs* a second opinion.

What's the best way to choose a consultant?

Sometimes it is difficult to know where to go for a consultation, but often an older gynecologist, well respected in the community, will be the best choice. He will have had extensive experience, and while he will have no financial interest in whether or not the patient has an operation, his professional pride will require that he give her his very best opinion in terms she is able to understand.

Of course, a woman may want to consult another gynecologist

recommended by her own physician. However, it's probably best that she avoid a consultation with a close friend or colleague of her own gynecologist. Unfortunately, he may agree with her doctor on the basis of friendship, when what the patient really wants from the consultant is a fresh, objective point of view.

Should a woman tell the consultant the whole story? Or should she let him make the diagnosis from scratch?

Medicine is not a hide-and-seek game where you try to test the physician's ability to ferret out your problems. You will save time for discussion if you frankly tell the consultant why you are seeing him, the concerns you have about the treatment or operation that has been recommended, and request that he give you his own candid opinion. Women must understand that medicine is not an algebraic equation, and a consultant is often not in the same position to evaluate your problem as your personal physician, who has been seeing you over a number of years.

Take, for example, the problem of irregular, or dysfunctional, bleeding. Suppose your gynecologist has watched you have this problem over many years. He has watched your bleeding gradually increase, and he can predict from your personality type and some of the tensions in your life that you may be a poor ovulator and that this problem is going to continue over the next ten or fifteen years of your menstrual life. He might, therefore, feel that the quality of your life would be increased if you were to have a hysterectomy. A consultant, on the other hand, would find an entirely normal uterus, and if you did not explain to him in detail the exact characteristics of your menstrual problems, he might not be able to understand that the hysterectomy is really indicated.

The same can be true concerning a sterilization procedure. Your own obstetrician may have observed the great difficulty you have had in your previous pregnancies, and indeed the problem of hypertension or diabetes which may become life-threatening if you were to become pregnant again. Unless the consultant understood this, however, he might say, purely on the basis of percentages, that there was no reason why you should not attempt to have another pregnancy, provided you stayed in bed, followed the doctor's advice, and essentially sacrificed a year to another pregnancy. On the other hand, if the consultant has the entire story from you, if you are candid enough to let him know all the facets of the problem, he can make a proper judgment, and at the same time allow you to discuss your thoughts, ideas, and difficulties.

The question of whether or not to have an operation for fibroids is another good example of how your own doctor might be better qualified to make a recommendation. He would be aware of the minor hemorrhaging the fibroid may be causing, and he may recommend a hysterectomy to spare you years of painful, debilitating menstrual periods, and to improve the quality of your life. But unless you give a consultant all the facts about your past history, he cannot make an informed recommendation or discuss all the aspects of your case in an intelligent manner.

Is it proper for a woman to bring her husband for a consultation?

I think this is quite proper and I often recommend it. Every woman has times when she would like her husband or lover to listen to what the physician has to say, particularly when treatment will involve problems of infertility, menopause, psychosomatic pain, and sexual disorders, where the partner has a vital role to play. I think obstetricians and gynecologists, in general, do not spend enough time with their patients' partners. They can be very important allies, and they can assist the patient in many ways, both physically and emotionally, in handling her illness.

I believe the obstetrician-gynecologists who take this family-oriented approach are the ones who give the best care.

What's the best way for a woman to open a discussion on controversial matters, such as abortion?

Such controversial matters often involve personal values, and here again it is important for the woman to speak candidly and to determine if she and the doctor have conflicting standards.

She should not allow herself to be intimidated or distracted from an open and thorough discussion of her doctor's point of view. This information is her right. She should simply say, "I want to talk to you about these particular problems." If the doctor's response is prejudiced or unsatisfactory, the woman should seek another physician.

In addition to abortion, are there other ethical issues that can divide doctor and patient?

Most often these involve contraception, sterilization, artificial insemination.

There are many physicians, the majority of whom are Catholic, who feel very strongly that sterilization is never indicated. If a woman has such a doctor, even though she may be extremely fond of him, have great confidence in him, and wish to continue under his general care, I believe it is proper for her to go to someone else to have a sterilization performed, if that is what she sincerely wants.

Artificial insemination is another area of conflict with both moral and legal ramifications. Some physicians today are concerned that they may be sued later for performing artificial insemination. Others feel the procedure should not be done for religious reasons, while still others have had some unhappy experiences in which the husband has rejected the child, knowing it was not his.

Again, a frank discussion is extremely important if you are going to receive maximum help from your obstetrician-gynecologist. You must be candid about your desires and feelings, and you must give the physician an opportunity to present his views. Then you are able to make a truly informed decision, even if that decision involves obtaining the services of another doctor.

Some of us are frustrated by the wall of assistants surrounding a doctor. What advice can you give about getting through to a physician who seems inaccessible?

When calling a doctor, the first thing to do is state your problem, briefly and clearly, to the person who answers the phone. Say, "This is Sally Jones, and I have a terrible vaginal infection, or unusual bleeding, or whatever." A lot of women won't tell their problem to the nurse, and this is a big mistake. The nurse will tell you if she feels she can answer the question or if she must refer you to the physician. One of the best ways to get many questions answered or to get through to the physician if you need him quickly is to explain the situation to the nurse.

Even if you are not having an emergency, you should tell the nurse why you are calling. Then indicate when and where the doctor can return the call. I have patients who leave a message that between such and such a time they will be at this phone, and between such and such a time they will be at that phone. Then I know where to reach them.

If you could describe a model patient, what would she be like?

She would be particularly observant about her own body and aware of any subtle changes in its function. She would also be able to articulate her concerns and observations to her physicians. Such a woman would often be truly helpful in making her own diagnosis.

I can tell you of one woman, age forty-five, who had chronic cystic mastitis, which is enlargement of the milk ducts in the breast.

This patient was particularly careful in learning how the enlarged ducts felt in each part of her breast, and when she noticed a small nodule that had not been present before, she went to a doctor. He diagnosed her problem as an extension of her chronic cystic mastitis, and, indeed, the odds were very much in favor of his being correct. She felt certain, however, that this lump was different, and she came to see me.

She was so sincere and described so distinctly the sensation of how this nodule felt that I believed it was important that we obtain a mammogram. We found this patient did, indeed, have early breast cancer, and thanks to her own careful observations she stands an excellent chance of recovery.

Another patient had complained to several physicians that her clothes were becoming somewhat tight. They assumed she had been overeating, a natural assumption, and instructed her in diet and nutrition. But this patient was certain her eating habits had not changed, and she finally insisted that her general practitioner take this complaint seriously. He referred her for consultation, and we found the patient had a fairly large ovarian cyst of borderline malignancy. When the cyst was surgically removed, the patient was totally cured. Fortunately, she had not accepted the simple explanation that she was gaining weight. She knew what she felt, and she was articulate enough to explain to the physician that there was a problem.

I could go on and on regarding how important patients are in their own diagnosis.

Another woman, for instance, described very subtle differences in her bowel movements which made possible early diagnosis of rectal cancer. And one thoughtful, articulate pregnant woman, who had had a previous cesarean section, described a tearing sensation in her abdomen which signaled an impending rupture of her uterus. Another cesarean was immediately performed, and her observation saved the life of her baby.

What makes for a difficult patient?

The most difficult patient is one who does not tell you the whole truth, withholding information that affects the outcome of treatment. Let me tell you about one young woman whose deception could have proved tragic. This patient was twenty-one years old, and the first time she came to my office she was complaining of extreme pain during intercourse. I asked all the usual questions and was told by the patient that she had never been pregnant and had never had an abortion.

When I began the pelvic examination, the patient had a great deal of pain, and I found her right ovary was attached to her uterine wall. This is always a sign of trouble because the ovary is supposed to move freely so that it can discharge its eggs into the fallopian tubes. Since this young woman had no history of pelvic infection or venereal disease and since she had never had an abortion, I considered endometriosis the most likely diagnosis.

This is a condition in which cells from the uterus escape into the abdominal cavity. I explained my suspicions and told the patient that we would need to make a "keyhole" incision and look inside her abdomen using a simple technique known as laparoscopy. I also explained that we do not like to perform this procedure in patients who have had previous surgery or extensive infection, as there is danger of perforation of the bowel when the lighted telescope is introduced into the abdomen.

At this point she gave me a funny look and said, "Doctor, there is something I haven't told you. When I was eighteen years old, I had an abortion."

She proceeded to describe how she had gone to some back street somewhere in Puerto Rico for an abortion. She became terribly infected and finally went to two doctors in this country who were unsympathetic and told her that she got what she deserved.

Her problems were due to an infected abortion. She had adhesions from the infection, became sterile, and eventually we had to operate on her and remove her pelvic organs to make her well.

Had I performed these tests and introduced an instrument into her abdomen without realizing that she had had a terrible infection, I could have injured her bowel and caused extensive and life-threatening complications.

2

THE EXAMINATION

Many women consider the pelvic examination a degrading experience. Few things are more awkward or demeaning than stripping down to the shoes, climbing on a hard table, and spreading one's legs.

I realize that we are all products of our culture, of what our mothers, fathers, aunts, and uncles told us; but it's too bad that women are told as little girls that they should never reveal their bodies to anybody except their husbands. It's about time we got over this unwillingness to show our body to somebody who can help us take care of it.

There is nothing shameful about the human body, and many members of the younger generation are now realizing this. Many young women today don't want to be draped during an examination. They kick off the sheet or deliberately let it drop to the floor. These women are telling me, "I think my body is beautiful, and I don't need this darn thing."

I respond by saying, "I wouldn't want this sheet on me either." And I go on with the examination. I regard these episodes as a healthy sign of the times.

These women are the exception. Right or wrong, many of us are still embarrassed.

I realize this, of course, and I have even had patients who put the sheet over their faces. When embarrassment is a problem for a woman, she should try thinking of the pelvic examination in the same way she thinks of an examination of any other part of her body. Is she embarrassed when she has her feet or her teeth examined? Of course not. But she has *learned* to be ashamed of certain parts of her anatomy, and she can unlearn; in fact, she *must* unlearn because this shame can have tragic consequences.

I remember one woman who so dreaded the physical examination that she neglected a sore on her vulva for a period of three or four years. When she finally did see a physician, she asked for medication but refused an examination. Later it was determined that she had advanced cancer of the vulva, and it eventually killed her. Had she allowed an examination earlier, her vulva could have been removed. Not only would she have lived but she would have been spared a tremendous amount of pain that resulted from her disease.

Many of us wonder what the doctor is thinking during the examination.

Most gynecologists are not thinking anything sexual, I can assure you. The doctor regards the female body as an incredible biological system. He looks upon the vagina, the urethra, and the anus as perfectly normal parts of the body, not as a sexual never-never land. These organs have particular functions in regard to making love, having babies, and passing urine and feces. And that is how the doctor regards them.

Of course he thinks of a woman as a sexual being, but her sexuality is not usually part of the relationship.

What can you say to help a woman who fears the examination?

I would encourage her to express her fears to her physician so they can be discussed and she can be reassured. I would also advise such a woman to request that her physician explain every part of the examination before it is performed. In this way, she will know what to expect.

Of course, every medical examination has a certain element of anxiety, and it is understandable that a woman may be concerned about problems the doctor may find, especially if she has had difficulties in the past or if she has special fears, for instance concerning cancer.

At what age should a woman have her first pelvic examination?

If a girl has not had problems with menstruation that would bring her to a gynecologist during her early teens, she should start seeing a gynecologist around the time she first starts having sex. This is when she becomes subject to all the problems and difficulties of an adult woman. We will want to check her cervix for abnormal cells—especially if she has had multiple male sex partners, which increases her chances of developing problems. Thus it is important that she also begin to have routine Pap smears.

It is also around the time when a woman begins having sex that she starts to contract urinary-tract infections and begins to have various types of vaginitis and venereal diseases. She is going to need contraceptive advice, and she should come to her physician for that.

Just how important are routine examinations? We are now hearing that they may not be as worthwhile as once thought.

Periodic checkups are essential if a woman is taking oral contraceptives, if she has gynecologic problems such as endometriosis or fibroids, if she is postmenopausal, and especially if she is taking hormones or medication. Regular checkups are also important if a woman has a strong family history of cancer.

Even if she is the average patient with no apparent problems, a routine checkup may uncover some hidden problems. So I equate a routine examination with a good insurance policy. If nothing ever turns up, a woman may feel she is wasting her money. On the other hand, she may feel it's worth the time and cost to have the peace of mind. Either way, the checkup gives her an opportunity to ask questions and be reassured.

What are some of the hidden problems a gynecologist may uncover during a routine examination or checkup?

A woman could be unaware of painless abnormalities of the vulva, vagina, and cervix which are either cancerous or could lead to cancer. By finding these conditions and treating them early, the gynecologist can avoid more serious problems.

In routine checkups, the doctor may also pick up early stress incontinence in which the woman may begin to lose urine when she coughs or sneezes. Many times he can show her how to exercise her vagina and improve her muscle tone so that she will not lose urine at inappropriate times or later need an operation.

Through his blood pressure checks, the gynecologist might uncover undetected hypertension, which can also be successfully treated if found early. Or he may find cancer of the breast or ovaries: the patient stands a much better chance of cure if this is found early. In addition, he may uncover early diabetes, thyroid, or liver disease.

Of course, another advantage of the routine checkup is that the gynecologist is available to give the woman contraceptive advice, and he may even improve the quality of her marriage by discussing minor sexual problems before they become major.

How should a woman prepare for a gynecologic examination?

We don't like women to douche before coming for an examination, particularly if they have vaginitis. Douching will wash out some of the yeast or bacteria for which we will be testing.

This brings to mind a patient who traveled over two hundred miles to see me because she had a bad case of vaginitis and had been treated unsuccessfully by a number of physicians, one of whom finally referred her to me. She arrived in town the night before her appointment and took a soaking tub bath along with a minidouche to wash out her vagina. When she arrived for her examination, there was no way I could get the slightest clue to her problem.

Is it all right to have intercourse before coming for an examination?

The only time this is not wise is if a woman doesn't want the gynecologist to know she has recently had sex. I have found sperm in women whose husbands were out of town for extended business trips. These women might not have wanted me to know of their extramarital activities, although the findings would have been safe with me.

Why do some doctors overschedule their appointments so that two or three patients arrive at the same time? This can create a terrible traffic jam with twelve or fifteen patients in the waiting room.

If I were a patient, I would complain about this. While delays sometimes occur, there is no need to keep a large number of patients waiting around.

Women also resent it when a doctor maintains a string of examining rooms in order to treat four or five patients at one time.

That happens to be a very efficient way to work, similar, say, to making five apple pies at one time. It simply saves time.

It may be efficient, but it's also impersonal. How can a doctor concentrate on one particular case if he's running from room to room?

He is not exactly running from room to room. He interviews the patient, he makes notes about her, but then she has to undress and get on the examining table. Since he has other women waiting, he uses that time with them.

Most gynecologists can adequately examine four or five patients in one hour. This number will depend on whether the patients are returning for simple treatment or visiting the doctor for the first time and will require a detailed personal, family, menstrual, and sexual history.

Nevertheless, there is definitely a feeling of being on a production line.

While a patient is entitled to as much time and attention as she requires to have a thorough examination and to have all of her questions answered, women must realize the doctor does not have to spend hours with them to provide good care. If Mrs. Jones has simply come for her checkup and renewal of her medication, I can do a pelvic and breast examination very quickly. If Mrs. Jones says she has no particular problems, and her past history has already been recorded, there is no need to prolong the examination. But when I look her straight in the eye, she must tell me what's on her mind. I should not be expected to have to coax this information out of her, although I will do my best to gain her confidence.

What should a thorough examination include?

If this is a woman's first visit to a particular physician, the examination should begin with a careful interview by the doctor of her health history. Does she or any member of her family have hypertension, diabetes, or cancer? Have her menstrual periods been regular? What have been her special problem areas?

Next the doctor will probably record her weight, height, and blood pressure measurements and check her heart, lungs, and thyroid. These things are all part of good general medicine.

The obstetrician-gynecologist is concerned with a woman's total health because any special problems she may have will affect the type of care and medication he will prescribe. He may also ask her to complete a general health questionnaire.

When I see a patient for the first time, I also look closely at her face. Does she have excessive facial hair? Is she producing enough estrogen or too much androgen, or male hormones? I sometimes recommend that the woman have electrolysis to remove excessive facial hair if the problem does not require hormone treatment and the woman is bothered by it. I caution her, however, that electrolysis must be done carefully and the hair root itself must be killed. Otherwise the hair will grow back.

Continuing the examination, I also learn something about the patient's personality by whether or not she looks me in the eye. And I examine her teeth and gums to determine, not only if she has periodontal disease, but how well she takes care of herself.

Next I will ask how she is getting along sexually. It is extremely important that women learn to expect their gynecologist to take an adequate sexual history.

What kind of questions do you ask about sex?

Basically I ask if there are problems she wishes to discuss. When I am examining a young girl and I don't know if she has begun intercourse yet, I simply ask: "Have you begun intercourse?" This is a very straightforward question, and I usually get a straightforward answer. If she says yes, then I ask her what kind of contraceptives she is using, and this again is a nonthreatening sort of question. Many times this is what the patient was hoping I would ask because she really wanted to have some contraceptive advice and was glad I brought it up.

To an older woman, I merely say, "Are you having intercourse at the present time?" Again, I'll get a fairly straightforward answer. To a married woman I'll ask, "How frequently are you having intercourse? Are you orgasmic? What percentage of the time? Do you have adequate vaginal lubrication? Are there particular problems you'd like to discuss?"

I always tell patients that I feel very comfortable talking about sexuality and I want them to feel free to bring up any particular problems on their mind. Once we have had this conversation, I go on to the breast examination.

Here again, some women can be embarrassed about having a strange man examine their breasts.

Then they should understand that when a doctor examines their breasts he is thinking about two things: fat and glands. He considers the breast a natural, functional part of the body, just like the hands or the arms. There is no sexuality involved in the examination. It's not the sort of thing he is going to get an erection from or fantasize about. So the patient should not worry about what the doctor is thinking.

What should a good breast examination include?

I believe that every breast examination should include a do-it-yourself lesson on self-examination, and every woman should insist that her doctor give her this type of information. It is not enough to hand a patient a booklet describing the technique. The woman must be taught on a personal basis, using her own hand to become familiar with the normal feel of her breasts.

I explain to patients that self-examination should be performed at the same time every month because the breast goes through normal monthly changes. The best time is probably one week after the cessation of menstruation, when the breasts are least stimulated and therefore less full.

I also explain to patients that they are looking for *lumps*, not necessarily cancer, and I stress that most lumps that women find in their breasts are not malignant. These are often caused by fluid trapped in the ducts (these lumps are known as cysts) or by fibrous tissue similar to scars on the skin.

During the first part of the self-examination, the woman should stand in front of a mirror looking for bulges in the breasts or for puckering of the skin. Then she should squeeze each nipple. Any milky discharge or bloodstained secretion from a nipple, or any sore on the nipple, should be brought to the attention of a physician. These things are not necessarily cancerous.

Next the woman should lie on a bed or recline in a tub, raising one arm over her head to examine the breast on that side. With the fingers of the opposite hand, she should gently feel in small circles for thickening or lumps.

She may find some glands in the breast which cause a lumpy feeling; this is normal—provided the lumps are symmetrical. If a lump, or series of lumps, is felt in one particular region in one breast, it should be compared with the same region in the other breast. If a woman examines herself frequently, she will be able to recognize any changes or suspicious signs, such as a distinct, single tumor.

Most of us dread examining our own breasts. We are frightened of what we may find. There is such a strong feeling of not wanting to know that the tendency is to rush through the examination or not perform it at all.

I can appreciate that, but no physician can examine a woman's breasts as effectively as she can. The doctor can only feel with his fingers, but the woman also has feeling inside her breasts.

The dread is normal during a self-examination, but the woman must realize that breast cancer is the most common cancer in females, and 85 percent of all cases are discovered by women themselves. So the woman has a very important role to play.

On the more cheerful side, once she has learned to perform the examination effectively, and she finds that everything is normal, there is always a great sense of relief.

Must both breasts be the same size?

No. Both breasts are rarely the exact same size, and the breast which is slightly larger will have slightly more prominent glandular tissue. One way to remember these differences is for a woman to keep a record as doctors do. She should simply draw a rough picture of her breasts and record how each area feels during the examination. The next time she checks her breasts she can make a comparison and detect changes.

If a woman does find a lump, what is the likelihood it will be malignant?

The likelihood is relatively small, maybe 20 percent. But every lump, no matter how harmless it may seem, should be evaluated by a doctor. Most often he will find it to be a cyst, fibrous tissue, or a general thickening or swelling related to the menstrual cycle.

What happens after the breast examination?
From the breast the doctor moves to the abdominal examination. While the patient lies on the examining table, the doctor feels her liver, kidney, and spleen. He checks for tenderness as he pushes down on the abdomen and releases his hand quickly. This can tell him if there is abdominal irritation that may be due to pus, blood, or infection.
Then comes the pelvic examination.

Many women have an internal examination every year without fully understanding what is happening.
That's because women don't know very much about their own vagina and pelvic organs. Every little girl feels her vagina and sticks her finger in it, but when her mother or her aunt tells her never to look at or touch her genitalia, the child learns that this part of her body is somehow different, and she never becomes familiar with her own anatomy.

Can a woman watch her own pelvic examination?
This is difficult to do because most of the examination is performed inside the body. I have, however, used a mirror to show a woman an outside sore on her vulva or vagina that I want her to check regularly. I have also given anatomy lessons to women who are interested. Using a mirror, I point out the various structures, including the lips of the vulva, the clitoris, the urethra, and the opening to the vagina. I am always delighted to do this because a woman who is familiar with her own pelvic organs is much better able to care for herself and to spot early problems.
Every woman should study her external genitalia with the aid of a mirror and should feel the various parts of her genitalia with her fingers. She should know the anatomy and beauty of her own body.

Exactly what happens during the pelvic examination?
The woman lies flat on the table, with her feet in the stirrups, and the doctor examines the lips of her vagina, then her anus and urethra. He is looking for irritations, infections, warts, hemorrhoids, and other unusual signs.
Then he uses a special instrument to look inside the vagina. This

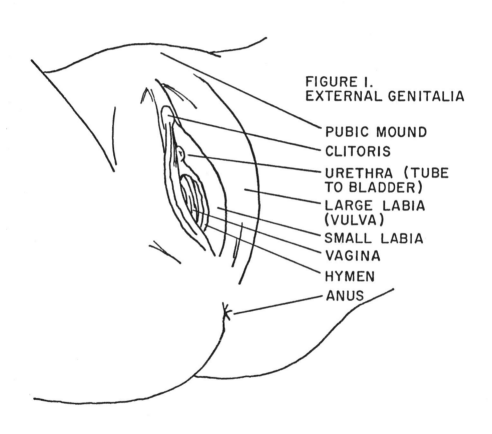

FIGURE I.
EXTERNAL GENITALIA

PUBIC MOUND
CLITORIS
URETHRA (TUBE
TO BLADDER)
LARGE LABIA
(VULVA)
SMALL LABIA
VAGINA
HYMEN
ANUS

instrument, known as a speculum, works like a duck bill. Once inserted, the speculum opens two to two and a half inches so the doctor can actually see the walls of the vagina, which are four to six inches in length up to the tip of the uterus.

If the woman is relaxed there is no pain. I recall one woman who would tighten up so it was impossible to insert the speculum. I finally told her I would just wait until she relaxed. She thought for a moment and replied, "I'll just pretend it's Robert Redford." Sure enough, the speculum went right in!

Occasionally I find a patient who is extraordinarily well relaxed, and she may even tell me what sensations she is having as I examine her. By giving me these critiques, these women have helped me learn to perform a more thoughtful, more gentle pelvic examination.

What does the doctor see inside the vagina?

The walls of the vagina should look soft and moist, much like the inside of the mouth. There should be no warts or polyps or irritations. The cervix, or opening of the uterus, should be clean and shiny and firm. There should be no ulcers or irritations. The vaginal secretion should be thin and whitish, which means it contains the cells which are normally shed from the vagina.

After these observations are made, the doctor will perform the Pap test to detect early cancer of the cervix. The Pap test is named after Dr. George Papanicolaou, who first realized that the cells from the cervix could be examined by special stains to determine whether a woman has signs of early cancer.

How is the Pap test performed?

With the speculum holding open the walls of the vagina, the physician can carefully examine the cervix. He places a cotton swab in the mouth of the cervix and twirls it in such a way that the cells on the inside are obtained for examination. This portion of the Pap smear is particularly important because some of the earliest cancers occur on the inside of the cervix. Then the physician uses a wooden spatula, like a tongue depressor, to scrape the outside of the cervix, applying particular pressure where the cervix has its opening into the uterus. He places these cells on a slide and sends them to a laboratory for special staining and diagnosis. The entire procedure is quick and painless.

Why is the Pap test so important?

The physician cannot tell, just by looking, whether a cancer is present. The cervix can appear entirely normal even though it may be the seat of early, or even advanced, cancer. The Pap test is the most accurate method we have for diagnosing cancer from living cells without actually having to cut off a piece of the cervix for examination, which is called a biopsy. There are many cases on record in which the patient showed no symptoms whatsoever, except for a positive Pap test, and these patients were found to have early, treatable cancer of the cervix.

Of course, if the physician is actually able to see a suspicious-looking area on the cervix, he will not only take a Pap smear but will pinch off a small sample of this tissue. This biopsy procedure is essentially painless since the cervix has few nerve endings. By fixing the tissue with a solution of Formalin and taking an ultra-thin slice, the doctor or a lab technician can use special staining techniques, look under the microscope, and make the diagnosis.

What does the doctor do after he removes the speculum?

He uses a technique known as manual palpation in order to feel the uterus and ovaries. To do this he places two fingers into the vagina on top of the cervix and pushes it downward, thereby thrusting the uterus forward. Then, by pressing gently on top of the abdomen with his other hand, he can determine the position and size of the uterus. He can also determine whether the uterus is freely movable, as it should be, and whether there are areas of irregularity.

Next he uses this same technique to feel the ovaries. These should be about one or one and a half inches in diameter, except in the postmenopausal patient, whose ovaries should shrink to the point where they cannot be felt (or palpated).

Once this portion of the examination is completed, the doctor examines the rectum.

Why is the rectum examined?

By inserting one finger into the rectum and one finger into the vagina, the physician is actually examining both areas at the same time. He does this for a number of reasons. The rectal finger attempts to determine whether there are signs of rectal cancer or of internal hemorrhoids, infected glands or small tears around the anus, known as fissures.

This rectal examination also gives the gynecologist another opportunity to feel the uterus and ovaries, which the doctor may not be able to do in the regular vaginal examination, particularly in women who are obese. This rectovaginal examination is also important

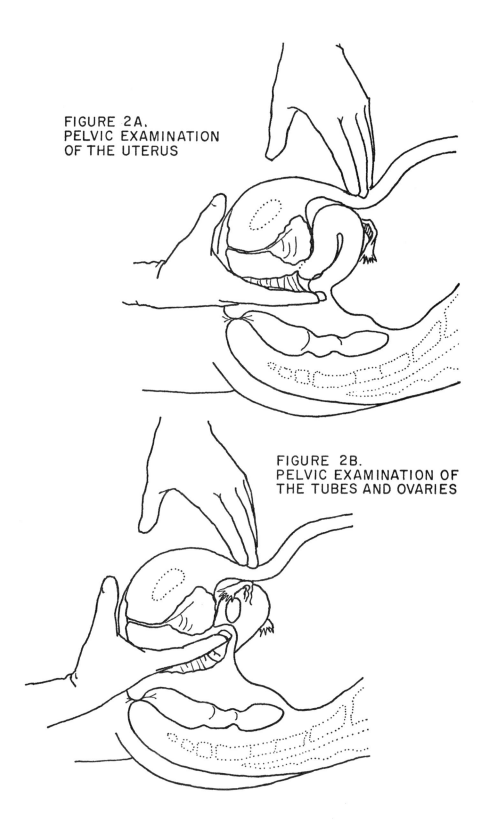

FIGURE 2A.
PELVIC EXAMINATION
OF THE UTERUS

FIGURE 2B.
PELVIC EXAMINATION OF
THE TUBES AND OVARIES

in examining virginal women. One finger in the rectum and one finger in the vagina is not nearly as uncomfortable as stretching a virginal vagina, and properly performed, it gives all the information that is required.

Why are vaginal examinations sometimes painful?

The pelvic examination is rarely painful, but when it is, tension is the most common cause. The muscles of the vagina are extremely strong, and it is difficult to penetrate the vagina if the woman does not cooperate.

Another common cause of pain is inflammation. If the vagina is infected or irritated, it feels like a bad sunburn, red and sore.

Occasionally there may be some pain caused by an unskillful or inexperienced physician. No two physicians are equally talented, just as no two people are equally adept at any skill, and for a doctor to improve his technique he needs to know how well he is doing. That's why a number of medical schools now have medical students examine female volunteers who evaluate and criticize the students' approach and technique. At the University of Alabama Medical Center, we ask our male students to perform pelvic examinations on their wives or partners or paid volunteers. These "practice patients" help teach our medical students how to perform an adequate, but gentle, pelvic examination.

Can you give us a list of questions to ask once the examination is completed?

If the doctor has uncovered a problem, you should be certain that you have the exact name of your condition and that you understand how it will affect your health. You should ask what types of treatment are available and how likely they are to help you. Always ask how long the treatment will take. Will it have to be repeated? How painful will it be? How much will it cost? What possible complications may develop? Are there alternatives to this treatment?

If medication is prescribed, ask for its name, how often you should take it, what it should do, how much it should cost, and what side effects it might cause.

How can a patient be confident her doctor is telling her the full truth about her condition? Are there occasions when you don't tell the patient the whole story?

I think a physician would tell every patient the complete truth if she were able to understand it at that time. Often, however, women are not prepared to take the sudden, total truth about a problem, and so you gradually educate them to it.

Take the case of a twenty-four-year-old woman who has extensive endometriosis, a condition in which cells from the lining of the womb are shed inside the abdomen, where they grow. Patients with endometriosis have bleeding inside their abdomen at the time of menstruation. This old blood has no simple way to be eliminated, so it adheres to pelvic organs with resulting pain.

This can be a very serious problem, and you have to make a decision. Are you going to tell the patient, "I'm sorry, but you may never be able to have children, the medical treatment may be unpleasant, and you may possibly have all your pelvic organs taken out before you are thirty?" It seems much more reasonable to discuss the disease and its ramifications and then explain the necessity for an accurate diagnosis. Occasionally a physician will think a patient has endometriosis and she doesn't. If he makes this error, he may set into motion a series of medical events which are unnecessary and unfortunate.

It is preferable, therefore, when one suspects extensive endometriosis, to look inside the abdomen with a laparoscope, which is a small lighted telescope that is inserted through a small incision made in the abdominal wall. This procedure eliminates the necessity to open the entire abdomen. Once this has been done, we can discuss the approaches we might use in therapy, and we try to assure the patient that together we will attempt to work out the problem in such a way that she will have the least amount of discomfort and the greatest chance to bear children if she wants them.

Let's take another patient, age fifty, who has advanced ovarian cancer. There is no question her chances for a complete cure are poor, but there is no point in my telling her at that moment that she may have so much swelling in her abdomen that she will not be able to have bowel movements and that we may possibly have to perform a colostomy. This may be the whole truth, but she does not have to hear it all at once. You tell the patient what you think she is ready to understand.

Sometimes our initial prognoses are incorrect. We have all seen the simpler methods of medical management of endometriosis prove successful, and a disease which we thought was going to progress rapidly and lead to infertility is abated, so that the patient is able to have several children. We have also seen patients who have extensive ovarian cancer respond beautifully to chemotherapy, then go on to have a reasonable and fulfilled life for three to five years.

It is, therefore, appropriate that we let the patient know that we are always going to be honest and straightforward with her and that together we will work as a team. It is certainly *inappropriate* to make long-term, guarded, or pessimistic prognoses, because many advances being made in medicine are allowing us to control these diseases.

But if the doctor seems to clam up when he discovers a problem, we often imagine the worst.

The physician who seems to be withholding information is sometimes mulling over the many aspects of the case. No matter what he finds, or thinks he finds, during an examination, the experienced physician remains calm and cautious, because he can never be completely sure of the outcome. We have all seen patients we were sure would be dead in a year and a half from cancer of the ovary turn out to have only an endometrial cyst or a benign tumor. We have also seen patients have lesions on the cervix that looked like cancer but turned out to be just a buildup of white cells. So it's important that the doctor remain calm and not paint too grim a picture, although he should certainly discuss with a patient the many possibilities of her disease.

How much should a thorough examination cost?

The cost varies, but I sometimes make the following comparison: How much does it cost you to take your car in for a 25,000-mile checkup? If you have a Mercedes or Cadillac or big Buick, it's going to cost you $150. If you've got a small car, it's going to cost you $75 to $80. Therefore, a thoughtful discussion with a physician, including a physical, breast and pelvic examination along with the necessary laboratory work, is really a bargain at $50 to $75. Just as the actual cost of the checkup of your car depends on how much labor is involved, what new parts are necessary and how complicated they are to install, the cost of your medical care will depend on the time a physician must spend with you and the tests he performs.

If someone comes in and is perfectly normal and just wants a Pap test and pelvic and breast examination, I can do that very quickly, although I would still go through some of the routine questions to make certain the woman didn't have a problem she wasn't aware of. But I would charge less because it takes less time.

Between visits to the doctor, how can a woman monitor her own health?

Mostly by asking herself how she feels and by understanding what is normal. Does her menstruation occur every twenty to thirty days? Does it last between two and seven days? Does she use from three to five pads or tampons each day? If these things are happening, she can tell herself she is within normal range.

Does she have stomach pain? Then she should ask herself if she is constipated. If so, she should try eating more fruit and vegetables. If she has a burning sensation when she urinates, she should increase the amount of water she drinks. Does her vagina feel irritated? Then she should wear pantyhose less often and use cornstarch to keep her vulva dry. If these problems go away, she doesn't need a doctor. There are many little things she can do to help herself.

Of course, we have already discussed routine self-examination of the breasts—a most important procedure.

Suppose a woman would like to examine her own pelvis. How should she go about doing this?

Self-examination is extremely difficult for a woman to accomplish thoroughly, although there are certain parts of her anatomy she is able to see and feel. She can certainly examine her vulva for sores, or lesions, by using a mirror. She can insert her finger into her vagina and actually feel the cervix, or tip of the uterus. She might even be able to move the cervix and to feel if there is any discomfort, which might be a sign of pelvic infection. But it would be impossible for her to palpate her own ovaries, as a doctor would, although she might be able to palpate the uterus to feel if it is enlarged. It would also be impossible for her to examine her own vaginal tube, from one end to the other.

Although a woman may purchase a kit for performing her own Pap smear, she is not nearly as likely to obtain as good a specimen for such a test as would a trained professional. Also, there may be hidden lesions which would be biopsied by a physician.

A woman can certainly examine her own rectum, but she can't push her finger up far enough to feel the cervix and the ligaments of the uterus. And it would be rather difficult for her to discover a cancer unless it was located right at the lower end, in which case it would feel irregular and hard.

It is possible, of course, for two women to examine each other, just as a physician does. Whether they can do it as well as a physician depends upon their experience. Even the average intern cannot perform a good pelvic examination at the beginning of his training. It's not until he is finishing his first year of residency that he is able to do a proper job, and the more examinations he performs, the more proficient he becomes. Two women examining each other could be the equivalent of the blind leading the blind.

3

MENSTRUATION

Why are so many women plagued with problems of menstruation?
Before I answer questions about menstrual disorders, I must explain
a few things. In the evolutionary history of human beings, menstruation did not occur very often. Women were either pregnant or nursing
their babies the majority of their adult lives, and this pregnancy and
nursing prevented menstruation from occurring. The menstrual problems that women face today are probably related to the fact that,
historically, menstruation was an uncommon event.

Also we must keep in mind that primates are the only animals that
menstruate at all, and we do not really understand why this is so. In
all other mammals there is no regular breakdown of the lining of the
womb at the end of the reproductive cycle. There is simply a periodic
shrinkage and regrowth. Recent findings indicate that human females
are biologically more similar to other animals in this regard than we
realized. Menstruation in humans does not involve a 100 percent
shedding of the lining of the womb as we once believed. We have
found, in fact, that only about 50 percent of the lining of the uterus
is lost in each menstruation.

How exactly does the menstrual cycle work?
The menstrual process is a marvel of timing and coordination. It
is controlled entirely by the ebb and flow of hormones that come
from three parts of the body: the ovaries, the uterus and special areas
in the brain.

The brain hormones known as FSH and LH (follicle stimulating
hormone and luteinizing hormone) signal the ovaries to begin to produce in appropriate sequence and amounts the estrogen and progesterone needed for preparation of the womb for the arrival and growth
of a fertilized egg.

Ovulation occurs about once every twenty-eight days when one of
the ovary's tiny follicles (or sacs) matures, and a ripened egg, about
1/200 of an inch in diameter, is released and sucked up by the
"fingers" of the fallopian tube. There are still many mysteries concerning ovulation (the eruption of the egg from the ovary) and conception
(the union of the sperm with the egg). The sperm have tails and are

capable of movement, but they are carried through the cervix, the length of the uterus, and down the fallopian tube by the movement of cilia, which are small hairlike structures, and by the contractions of small muscles in the uterus and fallopian tube. The sperm use their own locomotive power to drive themselves into the egg. This process is illustrated in Figure 3.

If conception does not occur, the production of estrogen and progesterone suddenly declines, and the uterine lining is shed as a menstrual period.

What are the most common menstrual problems?

Premenstrual tension, irregular bleeding and menstrual cramps are all common. Less common are problems of amenorrhea (no menstruation).

What causes premenstrual tension?

We are not really sure what causes premenstrual tension or irritability. I think it's important to keep in mind that the body is really programmed for a pregnancy to occur, and if this doesn't happen, it's almost as if the body is in great turmoil—trying to get everything ready for the woman to become pregnant during the next cycle. The lining of the womb which is partially lost in menstruation is immediately reprogrammed and rapidly rebuilt.

But problems can develop during the process. The estrogen, which tends to cause retention of fluids, and the progesterone, which causes the loss of salt and water, may be out of balance. The woman may have a retention of salt and water along with some slight swelling of the brain which may be responsible for the feeling of irritability.

So fluid retention is one cause of premenstrual irritability. Are there other causes?

As the lining of the uterus breaks down, it is also possible that slightly toxic substances are produced. These may enter the bloodstream, and cause some irritability in certain women.

Can these premenstrual problems be treated?

Because oral contraceptives prevent ovulation and change estrogen and progesterone production, they are one of the most satisfactory methods of treating both emotional irritability and the fluid retention which occurs in the brain and the lower extremities. The pill also causes the lining of the uterus to shrink, so there is very little menstrual

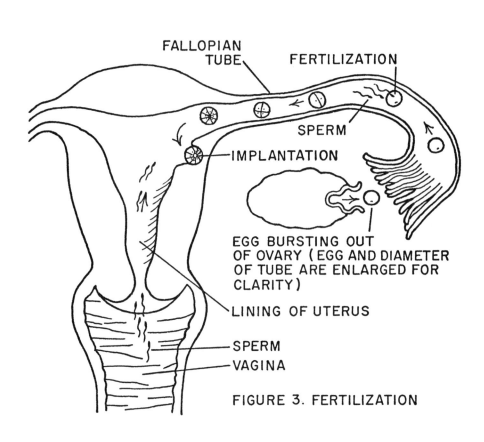

FIGURE 3. FERTILIZATION

bleeding and fewer breakdown products of the uterine lining enter the bloodstream to cause problems.

A perfect example of the effectiveness of the pill in these cases occurred approximately ten years ago when I was treating three patients who were close friends and who each had tremendous problems with premenstrual tension. One of the women said, "Frankly, I can't stand myself just before I menstruate. I know I'm nasty to my husband and to my children, but I just can't help it. So they all try to understand, and we have agreed that about five or six days of each month, just prior to my menstrual period, we don't communicate with each other very much, and I try to control my temper."

The second patient was extremely depressed and moody during her premenstrual days. She didn't want to be with people, her self-image changed, and she lost interest in her appearance and grooming. She also lost her sexual appetite. During this time, she would read a lot, but the books she picked were very depressing and often had psychiatric themes.

The third of these women developed a great amount of premenstrual fluid retention. She was a beautiful woman with olive skin and dark hair. Her lips were full, her body was supple and she was extremely proud of her looks, as was her husband. Premenstrually, however, her fluid retention was great. She had a slight swelling of her eyelids, a slight swelling of her ankles, and the seven pounds that she gained frequently went to her face.

I proposed to these three women that they take an oral contraceptive continuously for a period of six months; the results were remarkable. All three had a dramatic reduction in their complaints during these six months. The woman who couldn't stand herself became totally functional. The woman who was depressed and moody improved tremendously. She enjoyed clothes, went out and felt 75 percent improved. And the woman who had the fluid retention had a 50 percent reduction in this problem.

Suppose a woman suffers with these monthly symptoms but cannot tolerate the side effects of the pill.

Then we attempt to reduce the amount of salt and water in her body by restricting foods that are high in salt and by giving her diuretics and other special medications that increase the flow of urine. These diuretics are started about three days prior to the onset of menstruation and are continued until the second day of the menstrual period.

Do women who have had a hysterectomy but still have their ovaries continue to have monthly tension?

Often these women have a marked reduction in such problems. This has always been somewhat difficult for us to understand because, with their ovaries still intact, their production of estrogen and progesterone has not been altered—or so we thought until recent years.

Now we have come to believe that by removing the uterus we have possibly interfered with some control mechanism over the production of hormones in the ovary. What's more, with the uterus gone, there is no menstrual breakdown of substances that can enter the bloodstream and cause emotional irritability.

What causes irregular menstrual bleeding?

Bleeding problems most often come in two forms: breakthrough bleeding between periods, or excessive bleeding during the period itself. In either case it is important for a careful diagnosis to be made, and the first step is to determine where the bleeding comes from.

Often it is difficult for a woman who has irregular bleeding to know if the blood is coming from her vagina or from her rectum or urethra. This may seem elementary, but there are some women who actually bleed from hemorrhoids when they think the blood is coming from their vagina. Or the bleeding may be coming from a lesion or cancer of the vagina or uterus, and the woman thinks the blood is coming from the bladder.

If the bleeding is coming from the uterus, it can have many different causes, both physical and emotional. There can be abnormal bleeding from fibroids, erosion of the cervix, polyps in the uterus or cervix, cancer, or even emotional tension. So a woman who is having irregular bleeding, excessive bleeding, or bleeding in between periods must have a thorough examination, often including a D&C.

Exactly what happens in a D&C?

The term D&C stands for dilation and curettage. This is a minor operation in which the cervix, or mouth of the womb, is opened so that the physician can remove the lining of the uterus and cervix. By studying these cells under the microscope, he can diagnose the cause of the bleeding, be it cancer, polyps, or whatever.

Many women mistakenly believe that the Pap smear can diagnose all uterine cancer, but this is not true. The Pap smear samples only cells of the cervix and is unsuccessful in diagnosing cancer of the lining of the uterus, except in rare cases.

In addition to being used for diagnosis, the D&C also has a therapeutic effect on the bleeding. By scraping the lining of the womb with an instrument known as a curette, the physician removes any areas of infection and stimulates the healthy regrowth of the uterine lining.

Is a D&C dangerous?

The real danger of the D&C lies in the anesthetic, and that is why we like to perform this procedure under local anesthesia, usually on an outpatient basis. It is rare that I admit a patient to the hospital for a D&C under anesthesia unless she is an elderly woman whose uterus has regressed to the point where it would be difficult for me to adequitely perform the procedure, or unless the patient's symptoms require that I perform a more extensive examination.

Not only is the outpatient D&C under local anesthesia safer than one in the hospital under general anesthesia, it costs five to six hundred dollars less.

Still another danger of the D&C is perforation of the uterus, but this is extremely rare; it occurs most frequently in women who have cancer or some other abnormality.

Do young girls have different menstrual problems?

Often they do. Sometimes a girl is menstruating but not yet ovulating: she is not producing eggs, and she is not having a monthly rise and fall of her hormones. Her ovaries, however, are producing estrogen irregularly without producing the progesterone needed to control the growth and blood supply of the uterine lining. These young women may not menstruate for two months, then bleed for twelve days, then not menstruate for three weeks, and then bleed for six or seven days. In a thirty-day period, they may bleed for fifteen days. When the ovaries become exhausted and the estrogen production is shut off, there is a tremendous amount of bleeding because of the excessive development of the uterine lining and blood vessels. Nevertheless, such heavy menstrual periods in young girls rarely require a D&C. These girls have not really established proper ovulation and hormonal balance, and the doctor can usually treat them with contraceptive pills which contain estrogen and a progestin (the artificial progesterone that is present in oral contraceptives), or he can treat the patient with natural progesterone. These medications cause the lining of the uterus to regress and grow more normally.

Interestingly, all of these complex hormonal problems can be caused by emotional stress and physical fatigue.

How do stress and fatigue affect the menstrual cycle?

Periods of stress may cause a lack of coordination between the area of the brain known as the hypothalamus, which controls the emotions, and the pituitary gland, which controls ovarian hormones. When a woman is tense and upset, there is apparently a cross current between these two areas of the brain so that their functions interfere with each other.

That is why a woman who has irregularity of bleeding, who bleeds every ten or fifteen days, should look at her emotional life, because generally the problems are there. A good, thorough gynecologic examination is certainly in order, and many times oral contraceptives are a tremendous help, but taking a good long look at herself when she is having irregularity of menstruation is extremely helpful. In older women, too, erratic bleeding is often related to emotional and physical fatigue, which interfere with the proper rhythmical impulses between the hypothalamus and the pituitary. The result is a fluctuation of the reproductive hormones, leading to irregular menstruation.

I think we have all heard stories about women who began to bleed right after they had had some sort of shock—maybe their lover or husband died, or their parents—and they would begin to bleed no matter what time it was in their menstrual cycle. What happened was that their emotional center, or hypothalamic area, was suddenly stunned into inactivity. There was a sudden fall in stimulation to the ovaries, which then ceased their production of estrogen. And anytime you have a fall in estrogen, you are going to have bleeding.

When I was a physician in the armed services I saw the most dramatic illustration of this emotional type of bleeding. Whenever the Air Force pilots received their orders and were shipped out, almost all of the wives would begin to menstruate. It was while I was taking care of these women that I first fully realized the extent of the relationship between emotional tension and dysfunctional bleeding. I have come to believe that menstruation may be an excellent barometer of a woman's emotions.

How much bleeding is too much?

The normal menstrual period lasts from three to five days and releases approximately one to three ounces of blood. The average menstrual period requires a total of ten to fifteen menstrual pads or tampons. Menstruation is definitely excessive if it continues for ten days and requires the use of forty or fifty pads or tampons. This excessive menstruation will cause anemia, and it is necessary for women who have this amount of blood loss to take iron replacement, because they are losing much more than they could possibly derive from their diet.

How can a woman tell how much blood she is losing?

If the blood completely saturates one sanitary pad all the way through, she is losing 60 to 90 cc, which is almost 3 ounces—a normal month's quota. (A saturated tampon will hold only about one fourth to one third this much blood.) This means that a woman who is saturating many pads is losing a fair amount of blood. Of course, we can all lose 500 cc per month without difficulty. We can give that much in a transfusion, but if we lost this amount on a regular basis and were not taking iron, we would become anemic. Moreover, it's unnecessary to lose this amount of blood since excessive menstruation can be treated with progesterone or birth control pills.

What causes menstrual cramps?

Painful menstruation, otherwise known as dysmenorrhea, may have a number of causes.

The most common cause involves the production of substances known as prostaglandins in the lining of the uterus. The prostaglandins increase sharply just prior to menstruation and are believed to be associated with the contractions that initiate the menstrual flow. We believe, therefore, that excessive amounts of these chemicals cause cramps.

Menstrual cramps often subside as a woman grows older, apparently because the uterus has better coordination in eliminating the menstrual flow. Childbearing may also lessen cramps because the mouth of the womb has been enlarged and the uterus need not contract excessively to eliminate its menstrual material.

On the other hand, there are times when menstrual cramps may be a symptom of diseases such as endometriosis, fibroid tumors, or pelvic infection. That's why severe menstrual cramps should always be brought to the attention of a physician.

There is one good thing about cramps, however. They tell a woman that she is ovulating. If an egg is not produced during a bleeding cycle, there is no progesterone; if there is no progesterone there is no prostaglandin; if there is no prostaglandin there are no cramps.

What is the best treatment for menstrual pain?

While the most effective treatment is often the pill, which prevents ovulation, we believe that aspirin may also be helpful, and some women can take fairly large doses—maybe three tablets four times a day. The aspirin should be started two days before menstruation is expected and should be continued during the first two days of the period itself. The aspirin works by reducing the amounts of prostaglandin present. Hopefully, newer antiprostaglandin drugs will soon be available.

Sitting in a tub of hot water and reading a book can also be helpful, and we have always known that a bit of gin, vodka, or bourbon relieves cramps because alcohol changes the threshold of pain and possibly decreases the muscle tension of the uterus.

It is also true that some women find that masturbation or intercourse can be very helpful in relieving cramps. Masturbation and intercourse dilate the blood vessels, and the accompanying orgasmic response seems to quiet the uterine muscles.

Is it safe for a woman to have menstrual extraction so she will not be bothered with a period at a particularly inconvenient time?

Menstrual extraction, which is the removal by suction of the lining of the womb, is much too major a procedure to be used for this purpose.

I realize that menstruation can be a bother and that occasionally a woman might want to have the menstrual fluid removed before a particularly important event. But there is really nothing a woman can't do when she is menstruating. She certainly can make love, she can go swimming, she can dance, and she can participate in any sport. However, if a woman really wants to delay a menstrual period, the simplest thing to do is take oral contraceptives. She should start taking the pill seven days before the expected period and continue taking it for fourteen to twenty-one days.

We find that the majority of women who come in for a menstrual extraction are late with their period. They are afraid they might be pregnant, but they don't want a pregnancy test because they really don't want to know. So what the doctor is usually doing in a menstrual extraction is aborting the embryo during the second or third week of pregnancy.

What are the most common misconceptions you encounter with regard to menstruation?

The number of misconceptions that women harbor concerning menstruation amazes and startles physicians, who often don't explain this complex process to their patients. We doctors assume that all women understand this cyclic bodily process, but I find a great deal of misinformation, even among well-educated women.

Many women feel, for instance, that intercourse during menstruation is forbidden. Many will not allow their daughters to engage in exercise or wash their hair when they are menstruating. And in a study of one low-income group, some of the women even thought they should change their diet!

I have said it before, and I'll say it again: Women can engage in any activity they desire during menstruation.

You have mentioned lack of menstruation, or amenorrhea. What causes this problem?

I divide amenorrhea into three forms. The primary form involves young women who have not begun to menstruate by the age of eighteen. The second type involves women who have established normal menstrual patterns but who, for some reason, later cease to have periods. And the third type of amenorrhea occurs following use of the pill.

What causes primary amenorrhea?

Primary amenorrhea in young girls may be caused by failure of the ovaries to function properly. It may be caused by a pituitary tumor or by abnormal development of the uterus. Occasionally we find a patient who does not menstruate because she does not have a uterus or because she has inadequate or abnormal ovarian development. It is important that abnormal gonads be removed by the time the young woman is eighteen or twenty years old because of a small risk that malignancy may develop.

Amenorrhea may also be caused by obesity or psychic disorders, and here it is often difficult to determine which is the cause and which is the effect.

Anytime a young woman has not initiated menstruation by the age of seventeen, a physician should be consulted.

What is the treatment of primary amenorrhea?

Treatment will depend on the particular cause. If the problem is a pituitary tumor—an extremely rare condition—it must be removed. If there are glandular or emotional problems, they must be diagnosed and treated. If there are problems with the ovaries, estrogen may help. But if there are genetic problems, or if there are abnormalities of the uterus and vagina, there is very little we can do. The one exception is an obstruction of the vagina at the hymen which may be preventing the menstrual blood from passing out of the body. This problem can be diagnosed very easily by an internal examination. The treatment involves a simple perforation of the patient's hymen. The hymen, as most women are aware, is a thin membrane that surrounds and covers the opening of the vagina.

Why do some women suddenly stop menstruating?

If a woman who has previously been menstruating regularly suddenly fails to have a period for four consecutive months, we define her problem as secondary amenorrhea—unless, of course, she is pregnant. There are several factors at work here. The woman may have developed a hormonal imbalance so that she is not ovulating properly. Or she may have a pituitary tumor, or emotional problems which have interfered with ovulation, as we have discussed. Still other times, a woman may be entering a very early menopause, although this is very rare before the age of thirty.

We are also finding that secondary amenorrhea is sometimes caused by crash dieting. A woman may go on a strenuous diet to lose weight and her glandular function may be affected to the point where she stops menstruating. Women who run twelve or more miles a week may cease to menstruate; this should cause no alarm.

Treatment, once again, must be tailored to the cause of the problem.

You have mentioned lack of menstruation following use of the pill. Is this a common problem?

We define postpill amenorrhea as the failure to resume menstruation within six months after the oral contraceptive is discontinued. Fortunately, we now have a drug that allows the return of menstruation and fertility in postpill amenorrhea, but this condition rarely occurs in people who have had normal menstruation before taking the pill. Postpill amenorrhea is most common in women who have had previous menstrual problems and is often due to a sluggish interaction between the hypothalamus and the pituitary. If a woman has had considerable menstrual irregularity, she should probably not use the pill. Barrier methods of contraception, such as the condom, diaphragm, or jelly, would be preferable in her case.

4

SEXUALITY *

I've never known a woman who didn't have some questions about sex, yet few of us feel totally comfortable discussing the subject with a doctor. What advice do you have for the woman who is too embarrassed to open communication?

This problem might be overcome with a letter to the doctor explaining the woman's problems. She might simply say, "Dear Dr. So-and-So: I have certain sexual problems which I find very difficult to discuss in person. My problem is that I am not orgasmic, or I have pain during intercourse, or my husband is impotent, or whatever. I have an appointment with you on such-and-such a date, and I would appreciate it if we could discuss my problems at that time." This letter will inform the physician of her needs and will give him the opportunity to take the initiative in bringing these matters up.

Another way for a woman to obtain sexual information is through the feminist movement, or her local crisis center or community mental health center. Often colleges and universities have courses in human sexuality, and some of the larger churches offer sexual-marital counseling.

Are most gynecologists now trained in sex therapy?

Unfortunately not. Although medical schools have begun to include more information on sex in their curricula, this information has been slow in coming and most older physicians have had no training unless they have taken a continuing education course in recent years.

Nevertheless, I believe it is important for the average gynecologist to be able to take an adequate sexual history. He should be able to make the woman feel comfortable discussing her problem and offer some minor advice. Beyond that, his main function is to refer the patient to a qualified sex therapist who is trained to deal with more complex problems, such as sexual aversion or inability to reach orgasm. The therapist may or may not be an obstetrician-gynecologist.

I should also mention that if a woman's regular gynecologist or

* This chapter was written in collaboration with Juanzetta Flowers, R.N., B.S.N., M.A.

obstetrician does not regularly bring up the matter of sex in his discussions with patients, chances are he himself is not comfortable with this subject. Such a doctor may even impart his own prejudices or biases to the patient and not really be of any help with her problems.

How can a woman judge the capabilities of a therapist or physician?
It is always difficult for a lay person to judge any professional who is supposed to have specialized expertise. That's why one of the best ways of choosing a qualified sex therapist is to be referred by a reputable physician. Another way is to pick a therapist who has been certified by a reputable organization, such as the American Society of Sex Educators, Counselors and Therapists, or the Eastern Association of Sex Therapists. It is quite proper for the patient to ask the therapist about his or her education and credentials. Unfortunately, in many parts of the country it is possible for a sex therapist to hang out a shingle without licensing or certification.

Please explain the physical changes that occur during sexual arousal.
The first thing that happens to a woman during sexual arousal is that her breasts become fuller and her nipples more erect. The clitoris fills with blood and feels firm. The vagina also begins to lubricate, or literally sweat, coating itself with a fine film of liquid.

What causes that feeling of extreme pleasure and ultimate release during orgasm?
Our best understanding is that orgasm is caused by a buildup of nervous impulses during arousal and sexual stimulation. When these impulses are built to a very high pitch, the dam breaks, and they are released in a tremendous rush of current from the spinal column. Basically, what happens is that the clitoris withdraws slightly up under the clitoral hood so that it can no longer receive direct stimulation during this time when it is exquisitely sensitive to touch. The vagina balloons out slightly up around the mouth of the womb. Respiration is increased, and there may be a flushing of the face and upper torso, particularly in fair-skinned people. Then the muscles in the vagina go through rhythmical contractions which occur at .8-second intervals. Of course, there are various degrees of this sensation. A common misconception is that the orgasmic response is a twenty-one-gun salute, that the chandeliers are going to fall, the bed shake, and so on. This is just not the way that it is all the time. Although many women do feel as if every muscle in their body is tensed, that all the warmth and blood supply in their body is in the pelvic area and there

is a wonderful sensation of pleasure, other women have a less extreme response—perhaps just a feeling of warmth and closeness along with mild contractions. The intensity and duration of these .8-second contractions vary with such factors as mental attitude, concentration on intercourse, the security of the environment, the interval between sexual acts, age, fatigue, and general health. The peak of orgasm abates slowly in a woman. With repeated stimulation, she can become orgasmic again within a few seconds, unlike men, who have to wait for a few minutes, hours, or even days before they can have another ejaculation.

What is the most common sexual problem of the female?

Failure to have orgasm is probably the most common sexual disorder that gynecologists encounter—even though nature planned the orgasm as a necessary ingredient in all mammalian copulation. With the constriction of vaginal muscles, the orgasm has a definite role to play: to grasp the penis and stimulate it to the point where an ejaculation will occur. Nevertheless, it is unfortunately true that many women in our society have never experienced this type of response. Usually these women have had difficulty with their sexual development from childhood.

Sexual orgasm is a natural, pleasurable sensation, partially intended to ensure survival of the species, and orgasm will occur in all women unless they have an extraordinarily poor lover, psychological hang-ups about sex or a serious medical disability.

We know that women in primitive societies are regularly orgasmic unless they are fatigued, overburdened, have personal problems, or are on a near-starvation diet. Similarly, women in our own society may lose their orgasmic response temporarily when they are tired, depressed, or having marital problems. With appropriate treatment, over half of all nonorgasmic women can be helped by sex therapy.

What would such therapy involve?

Because many orgasmic problems in the female are really a matter of misinterpretation, the therapist should first try to determine exactly what the woman means when she says she is nonorgasmic. What is the woman feeling when she has sex? How does she feel afterward? Is she tense and keyed up, or relaxed with a warm sense of well-being? If she does feel relaxed, chances are she has had an orgasm and didn't recognize it because it was not the extreme response she thought it would be. Many times a woman's partner will complain she is not having an orgasm because she is not reaching the fevered pitch the

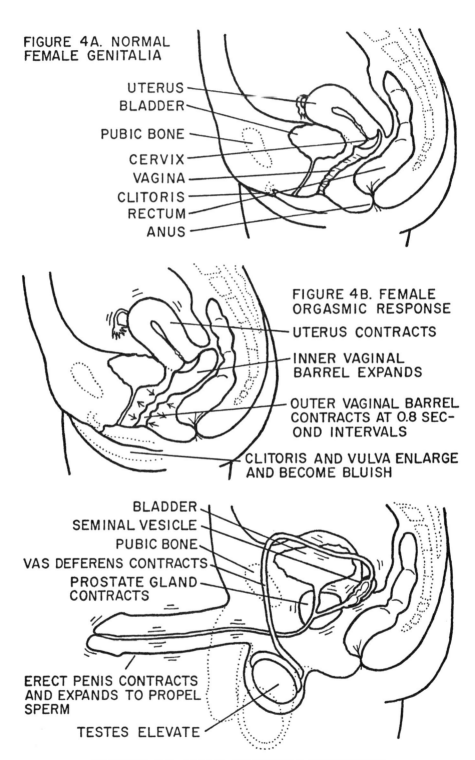

FIGURE 4A. NORMAL FEMALE GENITALIA

UTERUS
BLADDER
PUBIC BONE
CERVIX
VAGINA
CLITORIS
RECTUM
ANUS

FIGURE 4B. FEMALE ORGASMIC RESPONSE

UTERUS CONTRACTS

INNER VAGINAL BARREL EXPANDS

OUTER VAGINAL BARREL CONTRACTS AT 0.8 SECOND INTERVALS

CLITORIS AND VULVA ENLARGE AND BECOME BLUISH

BLADDER
SEMINAL VESICLE
PUBIC BONE
VAS DEFERENS CONTRACTS
PROSTATE GLAND CONTRACTS

ERECT PENIS CONTRACTS AND EXPANDS TO PROPEL SPERM

TESTES ELEVATE

FIGURE 4C. MALE ORGASMIC RESPONSE

partner expects. Such a couple needs to know that an orgasm is nothing more than a release of sexual tension through a discharge of nerve impulses. The orgasm is a physical sensation, but it also brings about an emotional peace or sense of well-being. So the first step in therapy is to make certain a problem really exists.

Once this has been determined, the next step is to find the cause of the problem. Is the woman unhappy in her relationship with her partner, or is she unhappy with herself as a person? Is she not allowing herself to have an orgasm? This is often the case in the nonorgasmic woman, and here professional help is often required.

On the other hand, if the woman feels warm and comfortable with her partner, she may only need a few suggestions regarding sexual technique.

What kind of suggestions?

The therapist may suggest that the woman fantasize during the sexual act or that she turn off her thinking processes and concentrate solely on how she feels while making love.

The therapist may also suggest that the woman masturbate on her own, so that she will know how an orgasm feels and will be able to recognize one when it occurs with a partner.

Sometimes a therapist will recommend the adjunct use of a vibrator. A vibrator is capable of making a woman orgasmic very quickly, especially if she fantasizes at the same time. In sex therapy, the vibrator is used with the nonorgasmic female, particularly one who has never masturbated, so she can learn what her orgasmic response is like.

One word of caution with regard to the vibrator: it is a rare partner who can compete with the vibrator either with his hand, with his penis, or even with his tongue. The vibrator provides the most intense orgasm possible, and a woman should not expect the same physical response with a partner. The vibrator can provide a woman with sexual release during the periods when she has no partner. However, one thing the vibrator cannot do is provide the warmth and tenderness of another human body.

What should a woman know about oral sex?

Oral sex is known as fellatio and cunnilingus. In fellatio, the partner provides oral stimulation to the penis. The practice is particularly useful when a woman is unable to have intercourse because of vaginitis or some infection. It is generally quite enjoyable to the man because he can become orgasmic with the sucking sensation. A woman may also enjoy performing fellatio on the male if she is sexually aroused, especially if she fantasizes at the same time. Many times a slight manual stimulation of the clitoris during fellatio will enable the woman, too, to become orgasmic.

What happens in cunnilingus?
Here the male orally stimulates the vulva and clitoris. This is a practice that most women can enjoy if the couple can get over their cultural hang-ups. But here again the practice may become addictive, for it provides a much more intense orgasm than intercourse can, simply because cunnilingus provides direct stimulation to the clitoris, whereas vaginal intercourse provides indirect stimulation.

Obviously, however, if a man or woman has grown up in a very conservative, religion-oriented home or considers all aspects of sex dirty, then oral sex will be considered a perversion.

The therapist will recommend oral sex only if it is compatible with the culture of the couple.

Isn't there a danger of acquiring VD of the throat through the practice of oral sex?
Definitely. If a woman's partner has venereal disease, she most likely will catch it, no matter what type of sex she is having—oral, vaginal, or rectal. It is important, however, if a woman practices oral sex with a partner suspected of having VD, that she have a throat culture performed by her physician. Obviously if a swab is taken only of the vagina, while the infected penis has also been placed in the mouth, the test results will be inconclusive. This is just one more example of the importance of open communication between doctor and patient.

Of course, if anal intercourse has been practiced, the test for gonorrhea should be taken from the anus. Otherwise the physician may miss the diagnosis.

What are other common sexual problems in women?
There is a whole group of problems which cause dyspareunia, or pain during vaginal intercourse. These problems may be physical or emotional in nature.

Pain may be caused by an infection of the vulva or fallopian tubes. The woman may have endometriosis or even very large fibroid tumors. She may have spasms of the vagina, known as vaginismus, which causes her to tighten up before intercourse because she thinks it is

going to hurt. She can also have pelvic congestion, which is an enlargement of the pelvic blood vessels, particularly the large veins beneath
the fallopian tubes. Here the woman may experience a sensation
similar to the feeling men have in their testes when they are unable
to have an ejaculation.

If all physical problems have been ruled out, a woman may have
pain during intercourse because she is not psychologically prepared.
She may dislike intercourse for a variety of reasons. She may feel she
is just being used as a sexual receptacle. If she had a fight with her
partner that morning, she may have no desire to make love that night.
Her vagina will not lubricate very well, even though she feels com-
pelled to have intercourse to keep a little peace in the family.

When a woman comes to the gynecologist with a complaint about
lubrication, it is extremely important for the physician to spend sufficient time discussing the personal factors in her life. If a woman
approaches these problems frankly and openly and does what she can
to deal with her difficulties, she should go ahead and use a lubricant
with no hesitancy. The contraceptive jellies or such lubricants as
K-Y Jelly and Transilube are excellent.

Lubrication is important because pain during intercourse can be
self-perpetuating. Once the woman becomes fearful of being hurt
during sex, she will become more and more tense. She will tighten
her vaginal muscles and be unable to lubricate. So it is important
not to allow the problem to go uncorrected. Of course, if a woman is
postmenopausal, her lack of lubrication may be related to insufficient
estrogen. This problem can be corrected by a small amount of estrogen
jelly applied directly into the vagina. If the lack of lubrication is being
caused by a medical problem, this must be treated. The woman should
refrain from sexual intercourse until the condition improves so that
she will not develop a fear that sex is painful.

What can be done for vaginismus?

When vaginismus is not caused by disease, and in many cases it is
not, the problem is probably psychological in nature. A woman who
wishes to deny entrance into her body unconsciously constricts her
vagina. This is a frightening situation because she cannot consciously
control it. The first step is to show the woman that the problem is
caused by an unconscious response. This can be done by using a
mirror and letting her watch the vaginal opening contract when it is
touched by a finger.

If the patient is willing to accept the psychosomatic, cultural, and personal factors that are involved, she should be referred to a competent sex therapist because the treatment is complicated and possibly long-term and requires good psychological support throughout.

Can pain during intercourse sometimes be caused by a vagina that is just too small?

It has been stated that the vagina can stretch to any size penis that the woman would like to place in it, and this is probably correct. The vagina can stretch without any problem provided the woman has had no serious birth defects or extensive surgery for treatment of cancer of the genitalia.

It is true, however, that a young girl who has a tight hymen or a tight vagina may have some difficulty during the early phase of her sex life. But with lubricants, gentleness, and time, the vagina can be stretched. If there is a significant problem, the tight hymen can easily be corrected with surgery.

It is extremely important, however, for a woman to allow the vaginal muscles to relax during intercourse, so that the vagina, being nothing but skin, can stretch. Skin is not unlike rubber. It can stretch a great deal—a characteristic that is quite apparent in people who have become obese and then lost weight. The skin, which has been stretched tremendously, actually sags because of the weight loss. So even when we do a radical hysterectomy in which we remove the upper half of the vagina, with time and gentleness the vagina will stretch to a sufficient size and length.

What can be done for pelvic congestion?

Treatment will depend upon the cause. Pelvic congestion, which is an enlargement of the pelvic blood vessels, may occur normally just prior to menstruation, and this is related to a fall in estrogen and progesterone. On the other hand, if an infection or a disease is causing the symptoms, these must be treated. When the woman is having pelvic pain with no sign of disease, this condition may also have emotional connotations and can often be improved with psychotherapy. For those women who can become sexually aroused but are unable to come to orgasm with a partner, masturbation may provide relief.

I should also mention that a controversial treatment for pelvic congestion syndrome involves hysterectomy, particularly in women who have finished their childbearing years. The theory is that if you remove the uterus, you have reduced the circulation that goes through the uterine and pelvic veins and therefore you relieve the patient of her pain. I am afraid, however, that many hysterectomies are performed ill-advisedly in these cases, because one cannot always be certain that removal of the uterus in the absence of the patient's ability to deal with her personal problems will relieve her symptoms.

Aren't there some male sexual problems that women discuss with their gynecologist?
   Yes. Two common problems are impotence and premature ejaculation.

What should a woman know about impotence?
   Women should understand that it is possible for every man to have periods in his life in which he is unable to have an erection. This temporary impotence may be due to fatigue, alcohol or other drugs, or simply due to the fact that the man's body has had enough sex for a while. These problems usually clear in short order.
   Impotence is divided into two categories: *primary impotence,* in which the male has never had a satisfactory erection with a partner; and *secondary impotence,* in which the male is currently experiencing difficulties but *was* able to achieve a satisfactory erection in the past. Primary impotence is very difficult to treat in that it has its basis in psychological hang-ups unless there are major endocrine problems. Secondary impotence can be more responsive to therapy.

What are some causes of secondary impotence?
   Sometimes the condition is caused by a physical illness, such as diabetes, mumps, or glandular malfunction, or even by radical surgery.
   Other times we find that the man is on medication for high blood pressure. This will interfere with his ability to have an erection and possibly with his sex drive. Just having this explained to the woman often helps her understand and accept the situation.
   Occasionally the man will have an abnormality in which a full erection is prevented by adhesions that run from the base of the penis to the tip. If he has not been to see a urologist, he should be advised that there are operations that can correct this problem.
   Secondary impotence can also have a psychological basis. Guilt, anger, depression, and even fear of performance are frequent bedfellows of the impotent male.
   It is important for the female partner to understand that an erection is an involuntary reaction. A man cannot will an erection, and a woman cannot demand one of her partner. The best way to handle this problem is with open communication. For if it is true, as has been suggested, that impotence is one way for a male to express his feelings

of anger, hurt, or rejection, the best way to correct the problem is to deal with these negative feelings.

How is impotence treated?

Depending on the cause, treatment ranges from psychotherapy to hormones, medication, diet control, and even a device known as a penile implant. This device is a collapsible silicone-rubber cylinder which is implanted inside the penile shaft and pumped up whenever an erection is desired.

While some interesting reports have come from China with regard to the use of acupuncture in the treatment of impotence, the most successful techniques in this country have been developed by Masters and Johnson. These involve a series of specific pleasuring exercises in which the partners explore each other's bodies with sensual touching and verbal communication. This treatment is best carried out under the direction of a qualified sex therapist.

What if the problem is premature ejaculation?

I think it is very unfair that premature ejaculation is almost universally defined in the light of the woman's reaction to the duration of intercourse. In my opinion, a man is a premature ejaculator only if he himself is not satisfied with the duration of his erection. As Shere Hite pointed out in *The Hite Report,* only 40 percent of all women are regularly orgasmic with penile penetration, so some men could remain firm and maintain vaginal contact for hours and their partners would still not achieve orgasm. That is why I feel it is unrealistic to describe the premature ejaculator in light of his partner's response.

If *both* partners agree that premature ejaculation is a problem, they should definitely seek therapy, because this problem is highly curable. And while they are waiting for the situation to improve, the couple might try using a vibrator or manual stimulation of the vulva and clitoral area to bring the woman to orgasm. A woman can have an orgasm in any manner she desires; it is not necessary for the penis to be inside her vagina. Her clitoris, which is the seat of her orgasm, can also be manually stimulated before, during or after penetration.

You seem to advocate masturbation as a technique that can be quite useful.

I have, indeed, found masturbation to be very helpful when a woman has no sexual partner, when her partner is incapacitated, or when her sexual appetite does not match his. As we have already noted, masturbation and orgasm can be helpful in relieving the heaviness that accompanies menstruation or pelvic congestion.

It is most unfortunate that our culture tells us that a woman should be orgasmic only with the penis in the vagina. Actually, intercourse provides less stimulation to the clitoris than any other kind of sexual activity, except anal intercourse, which provides no clitoral stimulation. This is no detraction from the maleness of the man or the femininity of the woman. It is just normal biology.

When does masturbation become harmful?

If masturbation is preferred to all other types of sexual activity, it may become a fetish and, like any other fetish, is not considered psychologically healthy. Masturbation can be extremely delightful when used in combination with fantasy, or when used to familiarize the woman with her own sexual capabilities and desires. Only the woman herself knows how much is too much for her.

We've all heard that masturbation could lead to insanity. What started this terrible threat?

In the 1800s it was thought that masturbation would make a person go crazy because young men and women who were in insane asylums masturbated frequently and openly.

When the Victorians, who felt they should be able to explain everything, began looking around for reasons for insanity, they noted the one thing that "crazy people" had in common was masturbation. With their own sexual hang-ups, the Victorians incorrectly concluded that masturbation must have caused the insanity, but the truth is that the insanity causes loss of inhibitions regarding masturbation. Excessive masturbation is a result, not a cause, of mental illness, and it is only today that we are finally beginning to dispel these myths—along with the other myths that masturbation is evil and sinful.

Are there other common misconceptions that you encounter with regard to human sexuality?

One common misconception is that women have a lower sex drive than men; another is that couples who have a great deal of sex early in their marriage will "burn themselves out." Still another misconception is that if partners really love each other, they will not have any sexual difficulties. And one more myth is that women must have an orgasm to become pregnant. Just not so.

Occasionally a man who is trying to initiate an affair with a woman will try to convince her that she cannot stay healthy unless she has sex. Of course, if she's sexually oriented anyway and she likes the guy, she may want to believe these things to give herself an excuse.

Another common myth is that men are always willing and able to have intercourse—or that if they are not it's the woman's fault. Men are *not* always willing and able. They have their periods of psychic fatigue, emotional problems, and other stresses that reduce their sex drive just as woman do. Actually there is very little difference between the sexual appetites of the male and the female. It's merely that society has placed many more restrictions on the female, causing more inhibitions.

These inhibitions are the reason many of us have difficulty communicating with our partners about sex. They may be the most important persons in our world, yet we may still feel reluctant to have a candid conversation about our love life.

This is very true and very unfortunate. Husband and wives can talk about the children, about the budget, about in-laws, friends, business, vacations, but when it comes to talking about their own sexual problems, this is a difficult thing.

One good way for the woman to open a discussion is to say simply, "I went to see my doctor, and he asked how I was getting along sexually. I told him I have these problems and he suggested I talk with you about it. He also said he would be happy to speak with you if you'd like." This approach allows the woman to move into the discussion in a relatively nonthreatening manner. After all, she is only following the doctor's orders.

Suppose a woman feels her partner is a poor lover.

While I generally feel that one woman's poor lover is another woman's Romeo, I also realize that some people are, indeed, clumsy at lovemaking. They are unimaginative in terms of creating sexual arousal. They do not use proper sounds, proper words, proper touching of the erotic zones, and they do not make the woman feel that she is wanted for herself, but merely for the sexual pleasure which she provides. It is up to the woman to show her partner what makes her feel warm and sexy. This is preferable to suffering in silence and turning her anger inward because of dissatisfaction with her partner's performance.

I also believe that a woman who feels her partner is a poor lover might do well to look at her own lovemaking techniques. Is she just lying there yawning, as some women have reported to me that they do? Or is she actively participating and doing things to provide her own pleasure?

Sometimes dissatisfaction with sexual techniques arises because there has not been good communication during the early months of a relationship. During this period the male partner will often do whatever feels pleasant and comfortable for himself. This is what comes naturally to him, and in the excitement of a new relationship, the woman finds whatever the male does exciting. She may not tell him at that point that there are certain aspects of his technique that she would like him to change. As the years go on, however, and she allows these things to become routine, she has only herself to blame for not speaking up.

A woman might be helped to open communication by obtaining some literature that discusses problems she is having and by reading the information together with her partner. She might begin, "Sometimes I feel this way," or "Sometimes this is a problem that I have."

One of the best ways to discuss any problem is to use what is called "I language," in which each sentence begins with the pronoun "I" rather than "you." A woman might say something like "I sometimes feel frustrated when we make love because I don't feel the way other women say they feel." Or she might say, "I am concerned about the infrequency with which we have sex," or "I really don't enjoy some of the ways we make love." A common problem that really bothers some women is the desire of their partners for sexual practices which the women find distasteful.

What kind of practices?

One practice many women dislike is anal sex. A woman may go along with her partner's wishes about this practice, but she is generally upset.

Then she comes to see me about some gynecologic problem and when I begin to talk about her sex life and I ask if there is anything she would like to discuss, she often hesitates. That's my clue to say, "Good Lord, we're old friends. What's going on?"

What do you tell a woman about anal sex?

Anal intercourse is exciting to some men because the anus provides more resistance to the penis than the vagina or the mouth. Other men desire sexual excitement by doing unusual or weird things. But the important thing to remember about anal intercourse is that the woman should be sexually excited and the man should use adequate amounts of lubrication to prevent pain. Ideally, it should be the final act of coitus rather than moving from anus to vagina, which can transfer bacteria to the vagina and cause infection.

Because anal sex is something that really turns me off, I find myself in the position of judging this practice on the basis of my own personal values, which, of course, I should not do. But the majority of women I talk with do not report enjoying this practice either.

I have found it is something that woman engage in because their partner wants it, and the first thing I ask is, "Is it painful?" Most women say that it is. Then I suggest that they communicate their feelings to their partner by saying something like "I enjoy making love to you, but not when you hurt me. I discussed this with Dr. Flowers, and he said I should tell you that making love this way really does hurt me." If the partner does not accept this complaint and still persists in his demands for anal intercourse, I would suggest that the couple seek professional help, because a woman is creating a big problem if she continues with this practice against her will. She will build up a great deal of resentment and eventually not want to have sex at all.

Don't men resent their partners' confiding such intimate details to the gynecologist?

I feel that some men are going to resent their partners' talking to their doctors about anything. These are men who feel insecure, who have a low self-image, and who are not comfortable with themselves. They do not want their partners to be discussing anything with anybody and definitely resent the fact that they have talked to another man about sex.

One way to handle this problem is to invite the man to come along for the visit to the gynecologist.

Do men and women often visit you together to discuss their sexual problems?

Men are coming in increasing numbers to talk with obstetricians and gynecologists about many matters, and this is something to be encouraged.

There is essentially nothing that an obstetrician-gynecologist would discuss with a woman that it would not be advantageous for her partner to hear, provided the woman is willing for him to hear it. There may be, however, certain details of a woman's past that should remain private, and her physician has an obligation never to reveal to a partner anything that a woman does not want the partner to know.

In years gone by, I used to think that men were coming to the gynecologist to protect themselves with regard to sexual matters because they were afraid the gynecologist would side with the woman and blame whatever problems existed on the fact that the man was a poor lover. And I have to admit that occasionally that did happen. But now with sex therapy available for those couples who need it, the discussion can include both a male therapist acting as an advocate for the man and female therapist acting for the woman. This type of situation creates much discussion and cross discussion which has been dramatic in its success.

Do women ever want to engage in sexual practices their partners find distasteful?

Men suffer from sexual inhibitions just as women do, so it is quite possible for this to occur. What the man might find distasteful can range all the way from intercourse in any other than the "missionary" position to anal sex. If this is causing a problem in their relationship, the couple should seek professional help.

What other complaints do men have with regard to their wives' love-making?

Most commonly men complain that their wives are nonorgasmic. I can remember so well a colonel in the army who was very upset that his wife did not enjoy intercourse. He wanted me "to do something," because he insisted it was her own fault. He said, "It couldn't be me because I can make any woman I pick up 'pop off.' "

What this man didn't realize was that sexuality is in the head, and lack of orgasm is usually not a physical problem. The orgasmic response is very primitive and is always present if a woman will allow it to manifest itself. Many times women are nonorgasmic because of the man. The problem is not always that he is impotent, but often that the woman is upset or angry with him.

Take the case of a husband who became infuriated when his wife did not hop into bed at his slightest inclination. It didn't matter what time of day it was, whether the children were around, or anything else. He would become furious if she didn't run and take off her clothes. When he came into the bedroom with an erection and promptly had his ejaculation, he couldn't understand why she did not respond just as rapidly as he did.

This man came to me complaining his wife needed circumcising to increase her sexual response, but when I spoke with the wife, she talked of her husband's insensitive behavior. It was not that she did not enjoy intercourse. She definitely did enjoy it when he would take his time and really make love to her. But most of the time she felt she was being raped. He didn't use a knife or a gun, but he held over her the fact that he supported her and that if she did not put out, he would go somewhere else. And that's really rape, too. It's the same principle as forcing a woman to have intercourse against her will.

You just mentioned circumcision of a woman. How is this done?

This type of circumcision involves removing a small portion of the covering of the tip of the clitoris, supposedly to make the end of the clitoris more sensitive to stimulation. Some doctors have reported success with this procedure; others have not. It is my opinion that the clitoris rarely needs to be circumcised to be responsive. Although the clitoris is the seat of physical orgasm in a woman, it is usually protruding sufficiently to be effective, if the woman is aroused.

The only time the clitoris itself might be deficient is if there are problems of adhesions from a former injury or extensive infection or perhaps from surgery for cancer. In this case, freeing the clitoris of its adhesions and allowing it to be more movable would be all that is necessary.

What other misconceptions do husbands harbor with regard to their wives' sexuality?

I have had husbands who were afraid to have intercourse with wives who had cancer because they thought it was contagious, and I have known husbands who complained that menopause was ruining their wives' sexuality—which, of course, it does not do.

I also had one husband ask me if I would give his wife testosterone, a male hormone, which he had heard would increase her sex drive. There are some gynecologists who feel this is true, and small doses of testosterone have been used somewhat successfully. This man was sure that was just what his wife needed.

This is something I am reluctant to prescribe because of the possible side effects, which can include facial hair, a deepening of the voice, and the development of other male characteristics. Moreover, I believe this type of therapy places the emphasis on the wrong area. Sex drive is a complex matter, and it responds best to counseling, where the relationship is treated rather than the libido per se.

Nevertheless, testosterone has been used for this purpose, and I recall one case where a physician-husband was secretly administering testosterone to his wife in an effort to increase her sex drive. The woman, who believed she was taking thyroid medication, came to see me, greatly concerned about the development of increased amounts of facial hair. Unaware of her real problem, we performed a number of tests and found a high level of testosterone, which seemed to indi- cate she either had a tumor of the ovary or problems with her adrenal gland. It was only when we informed the patient that she would re- quire some potent medication to deal with this problem that the husband came forward and admitted he had been giving his wife testosterone in an effort to improve her libido.

Can't some of these problems be due to a mismatch with regard to sexual appetite?

Occasionally this is the case, and it is an unfortunate problem when a woman who enjoys sex only once every week or ten days has as her partner someone who would like to have sex every day. It is equally unfortunate when it's the other way around. Occasionally, the problem may be due to differences in their biological time clocks. One may be a morning person, and the other a night person.

Most often, however, two partners who are mismatched with re- gard to sexual appetite are incompatible in other areas of their rela- tionship as well. They often have a problem in communication on all levels. One of them is holding back while the other is demanding sex as a way of gaining attention and satisfaction in a relationship that is not really satisfactory to either one of them.

The solution to this type of problem again requires the services of a marital counselor or sex therapist because the problem here is a relationship dysfunction.

What can be done when the passion wanes, when boredom sets in?

This is a very important question, and I believe that a couple who has become bored in the bedroom has most likely become bored in other aspects of their life, and they are just not willing to admit it. It's easy to complain about sex. It's easy to use sex as a reward, and just as easy to withhold sex as a punishment. Unfortunately, these things catch up with us in the end, so the most important thing to do to prevent boredom in bed is to keep the lines of communication open and to keep the relationship itself healthy and exciting. Of course, we can suggest certain sexual techniques to help put some zest back into a couple's sex life.

What kind of techniques?

These are essentially the same Masters and Johnson pleasuring ex- ercises which we have already mentioned. Each partner explores the other partner's body, excluding genitalia and breasts, in an effort to learn that the whole body can be involved in lovemaking. This is one way of breaking the pattern of a "kiss on the lips, a feel of the breast, and a dive for the pelvis" syndrome—a monotonous technique into which a lot of couples have fallen.

These pleasuring exercises are very reminiscent of one's early dating days when there was a lot of heavy petting before a couple actually began to engage in intercourse. Many older marrieds who are asked to employ these techniques react with giggling, but once they have begun to spend a little more time with their lovemaking, many report they are finding increased pleasure and are once again looking forward to sex.

What other sexual problems do women discuss with their doctor?

A problem which occurs frequently involves privacy. Sometimes when you are taking a woman's sexual history you find she enjoyed sex more before she was married. This is a common complaint. So I say, "Okay, let's talk about it."

We discuss how sex is exciting before marriage when the relationship is new and sex is something you are not supposed to engage in. You make love in different places—not in the same old bedroom— and all these things make for more excitement. Then after marriage, when children arrive, there can be the problem of privacy. My advice in that case is to put a lock on the bedroom door and teach the children about respect for privacy.

You can put a lock on your door, but when the children knock and you don't answer, they know darn well what you're doing.

Nothing wrong with that. It's healthy to let your children know that you and your husband love each other and express that love sexually. Just tell them, "When the door is locked, we wish to be alone." Sex is beautiful, but it's also private.

Suppose a woman is having an extramarital affair. Can she feel free to discuss sexual problems concerning a lover with her gynecologist?

I have had women who wanted me to give them approval to have an affair because their husbands were homosexual or impotent. Now that I am older, I think they are looking for permission from some type of authority figure, but I do not believe this is the role I should play. My responsibility is merely to point out the woman's options, to caution her with regard to venereal disease, and to provide any medical information which she requests. When I was younger, I felt that some women who were asking permission to have an extramarital affair were actually propositioning me.

Which raises the question, How much hanky-panky goes on in the gynecologist's office?

This situation is not very frequent, but men and women being the sexual animals they are, it is natural that some sexual interaction will occur.

There are women who proposition the gynecologist while he is performing a pelvic examination. The woman might make a slight movement against his hand, so that the chaperoning nurse will not be aware. Then following the examination, when the physician and the patient are alone, she will say, "You know, you stimulated me like no man has ever stimulated me before. It was just wonderful." Using this approach, she lets him know she would like to have intercourse with him.

On the other side of the coin, I'm afraid there are some physicians, hopefully in the minority, who proposition their patients. The physician will try to be as subtle as he possibly can. While doing a pelvic examination, he might stimulate the clitoris with his thumb in a sensuous sort of way, and he might tell the patient at the conclusion of the examination what an incredible woman she is and how she has sexuality coming from all her pores.

During the interview he might get up and put his arm around her in what appears to be a fatherly way, but which is actually a sensuous move. Or when he examines the breasts he may fondle them rather than examine them and remark on how beautiful they are. Then, depending on how far he can go, he might touch her leg with his leg, and perform any other sort of noncommittal act that could be made to seem accidental.

Women should be aware of all these things.

While we are on the subject of extramarital sex, please discuss the risk of venereal disease.

Venereal disease, which has acquired its name from Venus, the goddess of love, is defined as any disease that is transmitted through sexual contact. The most common types are syphilis, gonorrhea, herpes, venereal warts, and trichomoniasis, although we are also finding that the penis can be a carrier of other diseases, including hepatitis.

Venereal disease is definitely on the rise, due largely to the fact that people today are having sex with so many different partners. Years ago a woman would probably have sex with no more than one or two men in her entire lifetime. Today there are women who have intercourse with five or six men in one week, and this is not limited to prostitutes. Young women who live in communes or who have a poor self-image often have sex with many different men, and this increases their risk of acquiring venereal disease.

Of course, the best way to avoid contracting VD is to avoid sex with people you do not know well and particularly with men who have a puslike white discharge coming from the penis. Prostitutes have understood this for generations, and before they will have sex with a man they generally squeeze his penis to see if there is any pus coming from it. The average woman, of course, is not this sophisticated, nor does she have sufficient courage to do this.

Also, there is the added danger that gonorrhea may be a hidden problem. Many males—and females—can be carriers of the disease. Without actually becoming infected themselves, they can pass it on to their partners. It has been estimated that 80 percent of all women with the disease do not realize they have it until they have intercourse with a partner who develops symptoms of the infection.

What are the symptoms of syphilis in the female?

In the first stage of syphilis, a woman may develop a painless sore on the vulva or inside the vagina or mouth. Unfortunately this sore disappears in two to three weeks, so the woman might be misled into thinking she had a minor infection which has disappeared on its own. If not treated with antibiotics at this stage, the disease will progress via the bloodstream to other parts of the body and a low-grade fever and brownish-red rash will appear. Any rash which appears on the palms of the hands or the soles of the feet is particularly suspicious. If there is still no treatment during this second stage, the disease goes into latency. After several years, more serious symptoms will begin to appear, resulting in slow but steady destruction of body organs. Syphilis attacks the bones, the liver, the heart valves, and occasionally even the brain.

What are the symptoms of gonorrhea?

During the earlier stages, a woman may have a mild infection in her pelvis which may seem like an upset stomach. If she does not seek medical advice, the bacteria will pass through her uterus and eventually invade the fallopian tubes during a menstrual period. That is why the typical symptom of gonorrhea is pain or discomfort in the abdomen three or four days past a menstrual period. The discomfort is generally felt on both sides and is often accompanied by a mild fever.

If not treated early enough, this disease can leave a woman infertile by damaging the fallopian tubes. Many women who are now unable to conceive had such mild symptoms they never realized they were infected.

Other women will have more severe abdominal pain and higher fever, and they will see a doctor. Here it is extremely important for the physician to make a careful diagnosis of the pain. Is it caused by indigestion, appendicitis, or possibly pelvic inflammatory disease secondary to a venereal disease? Since pelvic inflammatory disease is generally not associated with a feeling of nausea, we can often rule out the possibility of appendicitis and begin proper treatment with antibiotics.

Of course, if a woman is engaging in oral sex, it is quite likely, as we discussed, for gonorrhea to affect her throat. With anal intercourse, rectal symptoms including itching, burning, discharge, and painful bowel movements may develop.

What are the symptoms of trichomoniasis?

Trichomonas causes a heavy, itchy, frothy green discharge which will go away by itself in time. The trichomonads, however, remain in the vagina and wait for the right opportunity to cause symptoms again. During the discharge period, the vagina is very red and sore and intercourse is painful.

How are venereal diseases diagnosed and treated?

Syphilis is diagnosed with a blood test, and gonorrhea and trichomoniasis are diagnosed with a swab specimen taken from the infected area.

Syphilis and gonorrhea are both treated with antibiotics. The treatment for trichomoniasis is an oral drug called Flagyl.

Venereal warts are treated locally with Podophyllin. At present, there is only symptomatic treatment for herpes.

What are some lesser known facts about VD?

There seems to be some confusion about certain diseases, such as trichomoniasis, Candida yeast infection, and herpes type II, which causes a fever blister on the vulva. All of these diseases may or may not be sexually transmitted. A woman may have Trichomonas in her vagina for a long time without symptoms until her body's resistance to the disease is reduced for some reason, and the organisms are allowed to grow and create problems—even though the woman may not have had intercourse for a long time.

The same can be said for herpes type II, which may be transmitted sexually or may have been living in the woman's body for many months before a drop in her immunity allows the herpes to multiply. While these diseases may initially be acquired through sexual intercourse, they may not manifest themselves until many months or even years later, so it is impossible to say how the original infection occurred.

What can you tell us with regard to sexual hygiene? Is it important, for instance, for a woman to douche after intercourse?

Different gynecologists have different opinions regarding douching. I do not believe that douching is a necessary part of postcoital hygiene. I tell women that sperm are perfectly clean and healthy and that the normal bacteria in the vagina will break the semen down into elemental products, so it is not necessary to douche. I particularly feel it is not necessary, or even proper, to douche right after intercourse. This is a time when the couple should feel warmth and affection and engage in communication and touching. This whole cycle can be broken if a woman feels she must get up immediately to douche because she is dirty.

Certainly the douche is totally ineffective as a method of contraception. Sperm enter the cervical mucus very, very rapidly, and the microscopic hairs within the cervical glands propel the sperm upward very quickly, so there is never time to douche before a sizable number of sperm are already up in the tubes fully able to cause a pregnancy.

So in my opinion, a woman should just relax. Later she will probably want to take a bath or wash her vulva because the bacterial breakdown of the semen on the pubic hair may seem malodorous to her, although some women do not object to this odor and think it smells nice. By this time the semen has become thinner and more fluid, and will run out of the vagina during a bath. Some women may need to wear a small piece of tissue or minipad in the panties, but many women don't need anything.

Suppose a woman is homosexual. Does she have special gynecological needs?

Homosexual expressions of affection cause no particular gynecological problems. A lesbian has the same needs as a heterosexual woman. When her sex drive is low or she is nonorgasmic, she becomes concerned. She can benefit from sexual therapy and should seek it if the problem becomes persistent.

What should a woman do if she suspects she may be a transsexual?

This is a very serious situation that must be handled with great sensitivity and special skill. The patient should first have a thorough psychiatric evaluation, and if she is contemplating a sex change operation, the decision must be tempered with time. The woman should undergo a period of very gradual transformation. She should be given large doses of testosterone which will result in the growth of facial hair, the deepening of her voice, and muscular development. During this transition period she should live as much as possible in a male environment and engage in the more traditional forms of male work. Sexually she will be put at a disadvantage because of her genitalia, but this is not an irreparable problem for a woman truly bent on a transformation. Although constructing male-type genitalia is a difficult surgical feat, there are some urologists who are willing to do the reconstruction.

Let's turn for a moment to the subject of sexual violence. If a woman has been sexually molested or raped, what gynecologic treatment should she receive?

If the gynecologist is a male, he should arrange for a female physician to see the patient, if possible. The examination should include antibiotics, tetanus shots, a vaginal examination to determine if ejaculation has occurred, and sperm studies, which may be needed at once. If the woman is of childbearing age, the gynecologist might also administer a "morning-after" type of contraception. This medication, however, should not be used on a regular basis because it causes excessive menstrual bleeding.

Because a rape victim has been subjected to a violent and sexual crime, the gynecologist should regard the rape as an emotional emergency and should serve as friend, counselor, and physician. He—or, preferably, she—should tend not only the patient's immediate physical needs but her psychic well-being as well. It is definitely not up to the doctor to make judgments concerning the crime itself, and the doctor should not make the patient account for her actions. It is particularly important for the physician to provide the opportunity for follow-up discussions since the emotional and sexual trauma may persist for many months.

Suppose a young girl has been the victim of incest. What can the gynecologist do to help?

By and large the gynecologist will rarely become involved in cases of incest unless the girl has been injured or is pregnant. This is usually because the wife and child are reluctant to seek help (I am assuming a case of father-daughter incest, which is by far the most common). Frequently the mother is furious with the husband and prefers to go to the police or to a social worker. This is unfortunate, because in many cases of incest there is a question of venereal disease or pregnancy.

If a gynecologist becomes aware of an incest problem in a family, he should strongly insist that they seek family counseling before irreparable damage is done to the psyche of the child. Incest is considered child abuse and is reportable by law in most states. A physician who does not report known or suspected cases to the local authorities is liable for judgment under the law—and so he should be.

5

BIRTH CONTROL

With all the new, improved contraceptives on the market today, how should a woman go about choosing one that is right for her?

There are many factors to consider: the state of the woman's health, her life-style and personal preferences, even her attitude toward abortion. Any woman who is definitely opposed to pregnancy and is not willing to consider abortion a backup for contraception should choose the most reliable method she can find.

The best approach is to discuss the pros and cons of the various methods of contraception with one's physician and then to make a thoughtful, informed decision. I believe that many times women don't use their contraceptives consistently or properly because they don't completely understand their use or because they were given a contraceptive they didn't really want in the first place.

Another important consideration involves the feelings and attitudes of the husband or partner. A woman is going to find it very difficult to use a contraceptive that is not satisfactory to him.

How do you go about advising a woman who comes to discuss contraceptives?

I find these women are of two types. One type wants to discuss the various possibilities, so we talk about the effectiveness and risks of each method. I ask them about their medical history to determine if they can use the pill. I explain the convenience of the intrauterine device and discuss the problems of cramps, bleeding, and infection, which may affect their fertility. I describe the use of the diaphragm and relate how some women find it most satisfactory while others consider it messy and inconvenient. Then I answer the patient's various questions so she can come to a decision.

The second group of women come in with their minds already made up. They know what they want, and it becomes a very simple matter to give it to them, provided there is no medical reason they should not have it.

Of all the contraceptives available today, which are most reliable?

Short of sterilization, the combination birth control pill of synthetic estrogen and progestin is most effective. These hormones, which are slightly different from the ones produced in the ovary, alter the production of gonadotrophins, or sex hormones, thereby preventing ovulation.

The combination pill has a failure rate of .1 percent when used with great care, meaning that .1 percent of the women taking this pill properly will become pregnant in a given year. This combination pill should not be confused with the all-progestin-type "minipill" with its failure rate of 2.5 percent.

Close behind the pill in effectiveness is the intrauterine device, otherwise known as the coil or loop. The IUD has a pregnancy rate of 1.5 to 3 percent.

Then comes the diaphragm, with a pregnancy rate of 3 percent when it is used with great care.

Which contraceptives are least reliable?

Contraceptive foams and effervescent tablets, with a failure rate of 5 to 10 percent, are unsatisfactory if used without benefit of diaphragm or condom. The withdrawal method, in which the man removes his penis from the vagina just prior to ejaculation, has a 7 to 10 percent pregnancy rate. The least effective method, in my opinion, is the "rhythm method," in which the couple attempts to avoid intercourse during the woman's fertile periods. Failure rates with the rhythm method range from 14 to 35 percent.

Do you recommend the condom?

In my opinion, the condom, which is a thin rubber sheath which fits tightly over the penis and collects its ejaculate, should be one of the foundations of contraception today, particularly among young people, because the condom serves not only as a good method of birth control but also as protection against venereal disease.

If the man uses the condom from the very beginning of each intercourse and withdraws his penis immediately after ejaculation, the pregnancy rate is below 5 percent. And if the woman uses an additional form of contraception, such as jelly or diaphragm, the failure rate is as low as on the pill.

Problems arise, however, if the condom is used in conjunction with the rhythm method. Couples who play safe periods and use the condom only when they think a woman is fertile are playing a dangerous game.

Pregnancy can also occur if the man does not wear the condom from the beginning of each intercourse. He should not wait until he feels he is ready to ejaculate, because he may unknowingly have already lost some of his most potent sperm.

Still another danger is that condoms, especially the inexpensive variety, may break inside the vagina. This problem can be solved with the new ruptureproof condoms made with a vulcanizing process. If the man will buy a good-quality condom and put it on properly, leaving a free space at the end so there is room for the ejaculate to accumulate, there should be no problem.

But many men dislike wearing the condom and are careless in its use.

It is true that the Western male, by and large, doesn't particularly like to use rubbers. Some claim the condom decreases their pleasure. I think this goes along with the macho attitude that a man should do what he wants, and if the woman becomes pregnant that's her problem. A certain amount of motivation is required for any contraceptive to be used properly. And that's why it is important that the feelings of the male partner be taken into consideration in the selection of birth control methods.

It is interesting to note that the Asian male has no objection to wearing a condom, and as many as 60 to 80 percent use this method of contraception. In large cities like Tokyo, condoms have been clogging up the sewage system, so the Japanese have made a biodegradable condom that will dissolve when it is flushed down the toilet.

So the pill and the IUD are the most reliable methods of birth control. It is ironic and frustrating that they are also the most dangerous to the woman's health.

It is true that the pill and the IUD both require medical supervision, and there are certain side effects that may make them intolerable to some women. But whenever we talk about the dangers of oral contraceptives and IUDs, we have to take into consideration the fact that pregnancy itself is hazardous and that it becomes more hazardous as a woman grows older. In a study of women from age fourteen to forty, it was shown that pregnancy is far more likely to cause mortality than taking the pill or using an IUD.

What are the different types of pills?

As we have already discussed, the most commonly used and most effective pill is composed of a combination of an artificial estrogen and another artificial hormone known as progestin. The second type of pill, known as the minipill, is composed of a progestin alone.

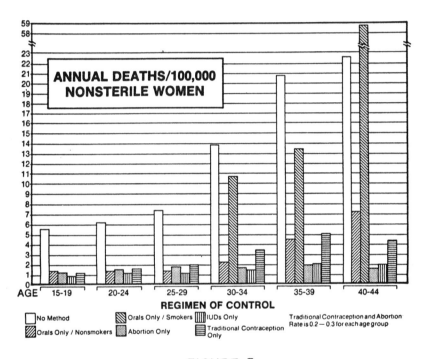

FIGURE 5

This chart indicates that oral contraceptives are extremely safe for all women until the age of 30. After that age, the use of oral contraceptives among non-smokers is much safer than a pregnancy.

How often should a woman take the pill?

The usual schedule is for the patient to take one pill each day for three weeks, then to stop for seven days. A simple way of remembering the three weeks is to begin and stop on a Sunday.

There are also twenty-eight-day versions of the pill, offering hormones only during the first three weeks and providing a pill without hormones during the last week. The purpose here is to keep the patient in the habit of taking the pill.

Finally, the minipill is taken every single day with no breaks.

How long does it take the pill to become effective? How soon can a woman be confident of not becoming pregnant?

The important thing to remember is that it takes at least seven to ten days for the pill to provide protection. So if you are going to switch from the diaphragm to the pill, you should continue to use the diaphragm for two weeks after you have started the pill. Then you're absolutely sure that your body has thoroughly suppressed ovulation.

From the condom to the pill it would be the same thing. You would continue to use the condom for two weeks after beginning the pill.

I hope everyone realizes that if a woman is on the pill regularly, it is not necessary for her to use a diaphragm or jelly or any other contraceptive during the five to seven days at the end of the monthly cycle when she is not taking the pill.

Many of us are frightened by all the publicity concerning side effects of the pill.

I think it is most unfortunate that there has been so much propaganda against the pill. Many women have developed unrealistic fears because of misinformation they have acquired through the media. The pill is a superb method of contraception for the majority of younger women. And since there are several different types of pills and dosages available, the pill can be tailored to meet the needs of most women. As figure 5 shows, the pill is far safer than a pregnancy and is as safe as any other contraceptive until the woman reaches the age of thirty-five.

Nevertheless, it is true there are certain risks and discomforts associated with oral contraceptives. The most serious of these include high blood pressure and a small risk of blood clots, stroke, and liver disease. There can also be minor side effects of nausea, fluid retention, headaches, weight gain, and minor bleeding problems.

A woman must weigh these risks and discomforts against any improvement she feels will occur in the quality of her life. If she places great value on being able to have a convenient, absolutely secure method of contraception, she may feel any risk or discomfort is of little consequence.

Who should not take the pill? What are the guidelines?

Oral contraceptives should not be taken by women who suffer from migraine headaches, liver disease, epilepsy, sickle-cell anemia, or blood clots. If a woman has a strong family history of early stroke, heart disease, diabetes, or hypertension, I feel she should use some other form of contraception. So should young women with irregular or problematic menstrual periods or individuals who have chronic emotional problems. Women over the age of forty and women over the age of thirty-five who smoke are probably better off with some other type of contraception.

Exactly how great is the risk of stroke from using the pill?

A study has been made in England by the Royal College of General Practitioners of 23,000 women who used the pill for varying lengths of time. Ten of these women developed cerebral thrombosis (a blood clot in the brain), as compared to three women in a control group of similar size not using the pill. These statistics seem to indicate that women on the pill are more than three times as likely to develop a stroke, but even ten out of 23,000 represents a very small risk. Women over forty who are on the pill are most at risk.

Is it possible for a pill user to protect herself from blood clots?

She can protect herself by recognizing early signs of possible problems. One of the symptoms that precedes cerebral thrombosis, or stroke, is tingling of the hands and fingers on one side for several days before the stroke itself. So if the woman has tinglings on one side or if she develops peculiar symptoms, such as headaches she hasn't had before, or shortness of breath, chest pain, blurred vision, or swelling in one or both legs, she should stop taking the pill at once and report the problem to her physician.

This was the case with a thirty-two-year-old wife of a physician who began to have tingling in the fingers of her right hand and who noticed that when she picked things up she would occasionally drop them or not be as coordinated as usual. This patient was intelligent enough to report her symptoms to her husband, who took them seriously. Appropriate tests were performed, and it was evident that this woman had had a very small stroke. The oral contraceptives were discontinued, the patient was given appropriate medication, and a major stroke was avoided.

Is it true that the pill can cause blood clots of the legs and lungs?

The data are very difficult to interpret, and the only valid study ever done on this question was performed in Puerto Rico in 1971. Ten thousand women were randomly assigned to either the pill or a mechanical method of contraception. There was an 80 percent follow-up on these patients and after eight years there were nine cases of blood clots in the legs among patients who were on the pill, and eight cases among those who were assigned to other forms of contraception. In other words, there was no difference whatsoever. There was also no difference in the incidence of lung clots.

Can the pill cause cancer of the breast?

Not as far as we know. All the studies that have been done, both in the United States and in England, indicate that the birth control pill is not in any way increasing the incidence of breast cancer. In fact, the pill, which inhibits the production of estrogen in the ovaries, may actually be helpful in reducing breast pain in a condition known as chronic cystic mastitis, in which numerous cysts develop in the breast because of excessive estrogen stimulation.

It is true, however, that if a cancer already exists in a woman's body, estrogen may make it grow more rapidly. That is why we never prescribe the pill for a woman who has a history of breast or uterine cancer. I must emphasize, however, that cancer in any other part of the body does not preclude use of the pill.

Why then does the pill cause some women to have pain in their breasts?

Tenderness in the breast may arise because of a general fluid retention that is associated with the use of the pill. These symptoms tend to occur during the first several months on the pill and usually diminish after the body has adjusted to the artificial compounds. If the pain in the breast persists for longer than three months, a lower-dose pill should probably be used.

Can the pill cause cancer of the uterus?

To the contrary. It is generally believed that the combination pills, which are presently available and contain both estrogen and progestin, actually protect women from developing cancer of the lining of the womb.

How likely is the pill to cause hypertension?

Although the development of hypertension is one proven complication of the pill, the risk is small. Only 5 percent of all pill users will develop this complication. Some patients have a tendency toward hypertension before they start the pill, while others develop the disease; but there is no way to predict whether it will occur in a specific individual.

Which women seem most likely to develop hypertension on the pill?

Most likely are women who have had a family history of hypertension or have had elevated blood pressure themselves. Women who have had problems of kidney disease or excessive fluid retention during their menstrual cycle are also more likely to develop hypertension on oral contraceptives. But women should understand that just because they have such a tendency does not mean they definitely cannot take the pill. I'm merely saying that they have to be more cautious and that they must see their doctor more frequently so that he can practice appropriate surveillance to detect early hypertension.

Even those patients who don't have a tendency toward hypertension can develop the problem—especially as they grow older. Pill-induced hypertension usually disappears within one to three months after discontinuation of the pill, although a few cases have been progressive. It is impossible, however, to determine if these patients would have had progressive hypertension if they had never taken the pill. Hypertension which occurred only during pregnancy is not a contraindication for pill use.

Is there a relationship between the pill and heart attacks?

Yes—among women thirty-five or older who smoke, are obese, or have high blood pressure, diabetes, or high cholesterol.

Pill users who have only one of these risk factors will have four times the likelihood of having a heart attack than women who do not have a risk factor. If a woman has two of these risk factors, then her chances of having a heart attack are about ten times increased, and if she's got three risk factors, her chances are almost eighty times higher. All of these factors increase the risk of heart attack whether the patient is taking the pill or not, but the pill does increase the risk to women past the age of thirty-five.

We have also read that the pill may cause liver and gall-bladder disease.

Since oral contraceptives are taken by mouth, they do pass through the liver, causing some slight increase in liver tumors. But these are extremely rare. Maybe one woman in 300,000 will develop this problem, and recent experience indicates that the liver disease usually disappears rapidly after the pill is discontinued.

In a small number of susceptible patients, the pill can cause gallstones to develop.

Why does the pill sometimes cause nausea and stomach upset?

The artificial estrogen and progestin in the pill must pass through the stomach and intestinal organs, which were not designed to receive these hormones. Taking the pill is quite a different situation from when a woman produces estrogen and progestin in her own ovaries. Then, these natural hormones exert their influence directly on the uterus and pelvic area without involving the stomach and intestinal tract.

To relieve the symptoms of stomach upset, it is often helpful to take the pill with an antacid or milk. If the symptoms persist beyond several months, the next step is for the physician to place the woman on one of the low-estrogen pills or minipills, which should relieve the discomfort.

Why do some pill users have bleeding problems?

Bleeding problems have different causes and different remedies. Spotting, or breakthrough bleeding, in the early part of the cycle is usually a sign of too little estrogen or too much progestin. The failure to develop menstrual periods at the end of each cycle also represents inadequate amounts of estrogen in most cases, but spotting during the latter part of the cycle followed by increased bleeding and cramps is a sign of inadequate amounts of progestin.

Although the solution to these problems involves the regulation of the hormonal content of the pill, patients should never merely double the dose they are taking without conferring with their doctor. This may upset the balance of hormones even further and cause more bleeding.

Neither should a woman discontinue the pill when these problems occur. She should see her physician so that the pill can be changed and these symptoms can be corrected. Many times the symptoms will correct themselves within three months. One of the major causes of unplanned pregnancies among pill users is discontinuation of the pill for minor reasons without seeking medical advice or using some alternate form of contraception.

Why does the pill sometimes cause menstrual periods to become scanty or even nonexistent?

I can't tell you how many women I've seen who were so concerned about their light menstrual periods or the fact that they occasionally missed a period that they presumed some terrible thing was happening. So they discontinued the pill, and many promptly became pregnant.

The major reason women on the pill do not menstruate at the end of each cycle is that the artificial estrogen in the pill is not nearly as strong as the estrogen that would have been produced by their own ovaries if they had been allowed to function. So the lining of the womb has not been sufficiently stimulated to develop and cause menstruation. This is not a bad thing. If one menstrual period is missed, this is perfectly normal. If a woman misses two menstrual periods, however, a pregnancy test should be performed.

Weight gain on the pill is another source of worry and frustration.

In some women there is an increase of five to eight pounds because of a slight increase in appetite or fluid retention. If weight gain is a problem, the physician can switch the pill to one with lowered amounts of progestin, which seems to be the primary cause. It should be noted that there is an equal number of women who lose weight on the pill. What's more, a woman can't predict in which group she will be.

How soon should minor side effects disappear?

Initial side effects, such as fluid retention, nausea, light-headedness, spotting, and bleeding, should generally disappear within three months. If these same problems develop later, they may not improve by themselves and it may become necessary to change the pill or discontinue its use.

Should a woman discontinue the pill if she develops headaches?

This depends on the type of headaches she is having. Women who have vascular headaches, such as migraines, should definitely not begin the pill. And those women who develop this type of headache while taking the pill should absolutely discontinue its use. Symptoms of the vascular headache include pain on only one side of the head. The pain is throbbing, progressing in intensity, and is sometimes associated with nausea, dizziness, visual disturbances, or a numbness of one arm or leg. Any of these symptoms absolutely requires that the pill be stopped and never used again.

Another warning signal involves numbness and tingling of only one hand or leg. This may be the start of a cerebral thrombosis (stroke), and the pill must be stopped immediately. On the other hand, if a woman has numbness and tingling of both extremities, this generally indicates fluid retention and is not a reason to discontinue the pill.

Nor is the tension (or nonvascular) headache reason for a woman to stop the pill. This type of headache tends to occur on both sides of the head, is nonthrobbing, and frequently radiates to the back of the head. Tension headaches obviously are not going to be relieved by discontinuing the pill because the tension is still going to be there.

Nor is a mild frontal headache, one that is generally related to fluid retention, a reason to discontinue the pill. Frontal headaches tend to occur only during the first one to three cycles on the pill. But if they persist, the problem is usually caused by an excess amount of estrogen, and the patient can be placed on a lower dose.

Why do some women on the pill develop hair loss and skin problems, such as acne or facial hair?

These women are unusually sensitive to the pill's artificial progestin, which causes some male characteristics. In general, these problems can be corrected by changing the pill and giving the patient a more potent estrogen. So again this is not a reason for the patient to just decide, "Oh, I'm not going to take the pill," or "I can't take the pill." There are ways for the physician to correct the problem, but only if the patient brings these matters to his attention.

What if a woman develops excessive pigmentation of her skin?

This problem, known as chloasma, or liver spots, is related to excessive estrogen but also to a lesser degree to the progestin in the pill. The condition is worsened by the effects of sunlight. The patient with chloasma has several choices: stay out of the sun and see if the pigmentation lessens, or go on the mini, or pure progestin, pill. If these measures are not successful, there is no choice but to discontinue oral contraceptives.

We have discussed the side effects of estrogen. What about the side effects of progestin?

This is another shady area where our information is inconclusive. There has been speculation that progestin may cause a reduction in sex drive, as well as feelings of depression or anxiety, or even acne and oily scalp. It has also been speculated that increase in appetite may be caused by progestin, but again this is difficult to prove. The most likely side effect related to progestin involves the development of very scanty menstrual periods.

What can be done for a woman who feels her sex drive has been reduced because of the pill?

Libido is a highly subjective matter that is very much related to many factors in a woman's life, including her self-image, how happy she is in the relationship she is having with her spouse or partner, and the tensions that are involved in family finances and raising children. When a woman is taking oral contraceptives and her sex drive is reduced, the first thing she should ask herself is, "Are there changes in my personal relationships that could account for this? Am I under too much strain at work? Do I have a feeling of guilt concerning the use of oral contraceptives? Is the reduction in my sex drive related to the pill or to other personal factors in my life at the moment?"

That's not to say that the pill can never cause a reduction of libido in some women. Occasionally it can, and this happens for several reasons; the pill reduces the reproductive hormones associated with ovulation, and it can reduce the production of the male hormone testosterone in the ovary. Women are usually surprised to learn that they are producing male hormones in their ovaries, just as men produce estrogenic hormones in their testes. It is this testosterone which may increase a woman's sex drive, so when the pill suppresses the action of the ovaries and less testosterone is produced, the sex drive may also decrease.

If this occurs, I think the best thing to do is discontinue the oral contraceptive and use some other method. In general the libido should increase within one or two months after discontinuation. If it does not, you know the problem was related to personal problems and not the pill.

While we are discussing change in sex drive, I should also mention that many women have an *increase* in their libido while taking the pill because they are no longer worried about becoming pregnant.

How long can a woman continue to take the pill? Should she give her body a rest at periodic intervals?

I do not believe in stopping the pill if patients are having no problems. Too many unplanned and unwanted pregnancies occur during the interval. As long as there are no serious side effects from their use, oral contraceptives can be taken indefinitely.

But isn't it dangerous or unhealthy to suppress ovulation for many years?
Actually the body is programmed for long periods without ovulation. Just look at our female ancestors. They did not menstruate more than fifty or sixty times in their entire lives. They were either pregnant or nursing their babies most of the time.

How often should a woman on the pill visit her doctor?
A woman should visit her doctor from one to three months after starting the pill, then regularly at six-month intervals.

Once a woman decides to go off the pill, how soon will her menstrual periods return?
Menstruation will return in the vast majority of women within six months. At the end of one year, 98 percent of all women who go off the pill will have had a return of menstruation.

Frequently the failure of menstruation to return occurs in women who have had irregularity of their menstruation most of their lives. They will continue to have irregularity after they discontinue the pill, and they would have had it had they not taken the pill.

If a woman has had perfectly normal menstruation all her life, the likelihood of having difficulty with the return of menstruation after she discontinues the pill is extremely small. A woman who has had problems with menstruation since puberty probably shouldn't take the pill anyway.

How soon does fertility return after the woman goes off the pill?
The return of fertility, or the return of the ability to conceive, is related to several factors: a woman's age, how long she has been taking the pill, and her own basic fertility. Some people are just more fertile than others.

We did one study where we followed four women very carefully after they discontinued the pill. We checked their daily levels of estrogen, their daily levels of progesterone, and their daily levels of all the hormones associated with ovulation. We found that all four women were ovulating within one month. But it took an additional three months until the lining of their womb was perfectly normal and the ovaries began producing normal amounts of estrogen so that they became fertile. The one woman in the group who was trying to become pregnant was able to conceive in the fifth month after discontinuing the pill.

How do you feel about giving oral contraceptives to unwed teenagers?
Different states have different laws in this regard. In Alabama it's perfectly legal to give a fourteen-year-old girl a contraceptive. But I always have a careful talk with these young people. I explain about the dangers of early sex with multiple partners. I discuss the possibility of venereal disease. I also discuss how sex can play tricks on them, how if they develop a sexual relationship with one boy, they are less likely to go out with other people and develop their personality. I discuss how they become more likely to marry at a younger age and how the divorce rate among the fifteen- to eighteen-year age group is about 60 to 75 percent.

I tell them how I see a number of fifteen- or sixteen-year-old girls who are pregnant and divorced. It's really a catastrophic thing. So I advise young adolescents to put their sex in the deep freeze until they acquire a certain amount of maturity. They don't always take my advice, so I never refuse oral contraceptives to a healthy adolescent. I think the use of contraception is preferable to letting her have an unplanned or unwanted pregnancy. Last year in this country one million teenagers between the ages of fifteen and nineteen years became pregnant. In the age group below fifteen years, 30,000 pregnancies occurred. It is safe to say that the majority of these pregnancies were unplanned and probably unwanted.

There are those who believe that the pill causes promiscuity. Do you agree?
No, I do not. The threat of pregnancy rarely deters teenagers from having sex. Over 60 percent of all teenage girls begin having intercourse without using any type of contraceptive. They just don't think they can get pregnant. So, pill or not, those who want to play around will go ahead.

I have found, however, that those girls who are mature enough to recognize the need for the pill are more likely to develop a meaningful relationship with their sex partner and are therefore less likely to be promiscuous.

What's meant by "the morning-after pill"?
This pill, composed of the synthetic estrogen known as diethylstilbestrol, or other estrogens may be used as an emergency measure to

prevent pregnancy after a single, unprotected act of sexual intercourse or rape. The pill, which must be taken for five days and within twenty-four hours after intercourse, prevents the implantation of a fertilized egg. However, the F.D.A. does not recommend diethylstilbestrol as a morning-after pill since abnormalities may develop in the vagina of female offspring. Thus the morning-after pill should not be advised unless it is understood that a therapeutic abortion will be performed if pregnancy occurs. Of course, this pill should not even be considered as a regular method of contraception.

Now let's discuss the second most reliable form of contraception, the intrauterine device.

The IUD is made of plastic with or without a copper or hormone-impregnated portion and is available in different sizes and shapes, often resembling thin wire springs. The device must be placed inside the uterus by a physician and removed when the woman wishes to become pregnant. We do not understand exactly how the IUD works, but we suspect that it irritates the uterine wall and prevents the fertilized egg from implanting itself.

Pregnancy rates with the IUD are low, only 1.5 to 3 percent.

What are the major complications with the IUD?

There may be complications of cramps and excessive bleeding, but infection is the most serious problem. Fifteen to 25 percent of the women who select the IUD must have the device removed, and those women who are able to wear it must check regularly that the IUD has not been unknowingly expelled. The advantage of the IUD, of course, is its permanent protection. It's always there, so you can't forget to use it, but it requires careful medical supervision, and there are certain side effects that may make the IUD intolerable to certain women.

Can a woman be fitted with an IUD the same day she goes to see her doctor about it?

Some doctors say yes, some say no. When the insertion is done during menstruation it is easier and one is sure she is not pregnant at the insertion.

Which women should not use the IUD?

Those women who have heavy bleeding, prolonged periods or severe menstrual cramps.

Can the IUD cause fibroids?

No.

Why do some women have excessive bleeding with the IUD?

We feel that truly excessive bleeding with the IUD is caused by a low-grade infection in the uterus which increases its blood supply. This situation is similar to when you cut your hand or have a splinter, which causes redness around the area. This increased blood supply is one of nature's defense mechanisms to overcome the infection.

Women who have excessive bleeding with cramps can try the new progesterone IUD, which causes regression of the lining of the womb with less bleeding. Unfortunately, the pregnancy rate with this type of IUD seems slightly higher.

Another type of bleeding problem sometimes arises in patients who have been wearing the IUD successfully for a number of years. This problem may develop because of calcium deposits on the IUD which damage the lining of the womb excessively and then break the blood vessels and cause bleeding. Other times, particularly in women over the age of thirty, the IUD will cause increasing amounts of irritation, to the point where there is a greater breakdown of the blood vessels in the lining of the uterus.

Of course, many women past the age of thirty begin to have variations in their hormone production with or without the IUD, and they can have increased amounts of bleeding. When the woman is wearing an IUD and this happens, we must remove the device and do a D&C to rule out the possibility of cancer and to remove any chronically infected material in the lining of the womb. The IUD can then be replaced in about six weeks, or some other form of contraception can be used.

Since infection is a common problem with the IUD, could you tell us some symptoms to watch for?

Symptoms include fever, chills, abdominal aches and pains, an odorous vaginal discharge, and, particularly, pain during intercourse, It has been estimtaed that a woman who has multiple sex partners has a five times greater chance of having a severe intrauterine infection related to an IUD than women in the population at large. This is simply because her vagina is exposed to more bacteria from different sex partners.

If the infection becomes extensive, so that the tubes and ovaries become involved, the IUD must be removed. The patient should be placed in the hospital and given large doses of intravenous antibiotics.

Otherwise tubal or ovarian abscesses may develop, requiring extensive surgery. When a woman is given an IUD, she should be told about the risk of serious infection, especially if she is having sex with multiple partners, because then the risk increases. This infection might later affect her ability to conceive should she wish to become pregnant.

Can the IUD damage the uterus?

Perforations have occurred with all types of IUDs. Often this problem is related to improper insertion, when the IUD may penetrate a bit into the wall of the uterus. Gradually it works its way deeper until it finally works through to the abdominal cavity.

If an IUD made of copper gets out into the abdominal cavity, the copper can cause irritation or damage to the intestine, and we feel that these IUDs should always be removed.

On the other hand, a plastic IUD without copper is not likely to cause irritation, so I personally don't advocate its removal. Now there are some women who get terribly upset that an IUD has worked its way into their abdomen, and they begin to have all sorts of vague complaints and difficulties, and eventually the IUD is removed. But removal in these cases is not something that is medically required.

Should the IUD be replaced periodically?

This depends on the type of device. The Copper 7, which is the IUD shaped like a 7 with copper wound around it, must be replaced every three years, the Progestesert every year. This is because the copper and the progesterone are dissolved by the body tissue, and the IUD loses some of its effectiveness.

Other intrauterine devices that do not contain copper or progesterone may remain in place for five or six years or even longer. If a woman is getting along well with an IUD, there is certainly no point in removing it.

How is the IUD removed from the abdominal cavity?

Sometimes by using the laparoscope we can make a very small abdominal incision to remove the IUD, and this is always the simplest technique when it works. To do this, the physician actually makes two small incisions. In one he inserts a small telescopic device (the laparoscope) through which he can locate the IUD. In the other incision he inserts a small instrument, or probe, by which he can manipulate and remove the IUD.

If it is not possible to extract the IUD in this fashion, we make a somewhat larger abdominal incision to get the job done.

How soon does fertility return after an IUD is removed?

Fertility usually returns quite rapidly, often within four to six weeks or even earlier. This depends upon how much irritation has occurred within the uterus, upon the natural fertility of the patient, and upon her age.

Of course, as soon as a woman has an IUD removed, she must begin another contraceptive method.

After hearing of the hazards of the pill and IUD, the diaphragm seems to me to be the safest of the reliable methods of contraception. Could you explain its use?

The diaphragm is a rubber domelike device approximately three inches in diameter. It should be covered with contraceptive jelly, inserted into the vagina, and placed securely over the tip of the cervix, or entrance to the womb, so that it acts as a barrier against sperm. The diaphragm is a superb method of contraception and the one that my generation used with no side effects.

With the advent of the pill and the IUD, the diaphragm declined in popularity. But now there is a trend back to this form of contraception and it is the third most popular method (after the pill and IUD), particularly among better-informed patients. I recommend it heartily for those women who are willing to use it carefully.

For the diaphragm to be successful, however, the patient must be motivated. She must not mind putting her fingers into her vagina, and she must learn to live with the diaphragm and accept it almost as a part of her body.

Of course, the diaphragm must be fitted properly so that the cervix, or opening to the uterus, is completely covered. Once it is fitted, the patient must learn to check the diaphragm's positioning. She must learn what the cervix feels like, and she must make sure it is covered with rubber each time she has sex. The jelly is most important; about one teaspoon should be placed inside the diaphragm so the cervix actually sits in this pool of jelly that contains a chemical which will kill sperm.

Why do some women have such difficulty learning to use the diaphragm?

Usually because they have not been given adequate instruction. One story that stands out in my mind involves a young woman who went to see her physician for a premarital examination. The young woman requested a diaphragm, and that particular physician was apparently somewhat bashful about diaphragm fittings. He performed a pelvic examination, wrote a prescription for the diaphragm size, and gave her a booklet, saying, "Read this, and if you have any difficulties come back to see me." The young woman obtained the diaphragm, packed it with her trousseau and planned to read the instructions during the wedding night.

The couple had a very big and very expensive wedding and reception, then flew to Bermuda for their honeymoon. They had a champagne supper in their room, and then the new husband went to put on his fancy pajamas and the bride went to the bathroom to put on her negligee and do all the things a woman does just before she is to enter the nuptial bed. Then she took out the diaphragm and read the directions. To her great frustration, she had tremendous difficulty getting the diaphragm inside the vagina. It was slimy and slippery, and she was on the verge of tears, exhausted from the wedding and all the anxiety. When she looked out of the bathroom, she saw her husband parading somewhat anxiously, so she decided to give the diaphragm one more try. Once more it refused to remain in place. Totally disgusted, she threw the thing away and promptly got pregnant.

What should *a doctor do when prescribing a diaphragm?*

When I fit a diaphragm, I do an internal examination to be sure the pelvis is normal. Then I insert the diaphragm myself and have the patient feel her cervix to be sure she knows what it feels like and can tell when it is covered. Then I have her take the diaphragm out and reinsert it, checking the cervix once more. I have her practice the procedure several times, with one of my nurses or female assistants helping her.

If she is having problems, I advise her to practice for a week and then come back to see me. In the meantime, her husband or partner should use a condom.

But the diaphragm is such a mood-breaker. It's a nuisance to jump up from bed to put it in place.

Some women avoid this problem by inserting the diaphragm every night in a bedtime ritual much like brushing one's teeth.

Of course, common sense should prevail. I remember one clinic patient, unfortunately not very intelligent, who had trouble with pills and trouble with the IUD, so we decided to try the diaphragm. We spent considerable time teaching her to insert it properly. Then, so there would be no confusion, we made it very clear that she was to wear the diaphragm every single night and that she was to take it out the next morning. In a few months, lo and behold, the patient was back, pregnant. We couldn't figure out what had gone wrong. How could she possibly have gotten pregnant? Finally a light dawned. We asked if she ever had intercourse during the day. "Oh, yes," she replied, "all the time. My husband works at night."

How long should the diaphragm be kept in place after intercourse?
Six to eight hours.

What if a couple wants to repeat intercourse within this period?
This is no problem if the woman takes proper precautions. She should check to make sure the diaphragm is still covering the cervix (because an orgasm from the previous intercourse may have displaced it), and then, leaving the diaphragm in place, she should inject additional jelly, using a special applicator. The diaphragm can be left in place and used repeatedly with additional jelly for as long as twenty-four hours. But the cervix must be checked before each coitus to be sure it is properly covered.

The use of the jelly with the diaphragm is so messy. Isn't there some more appealing system?
Researchers are working to develop a jelly similar to normal vaginal secretion. Instead of becoming sticky and messy, this jelly would evaporate just like the body's own vaginal secretion. Hopefully, it will be on the market before long.

Can the diaphragm get lost internally?
Absolutely not. The opening to the womb is much too small for a diaphragm to pass through, so it will always remain in the vagina until it is removed.

This is illustrated by the case of one young woman from North Carolina who was fitted with a diaphragm before going off to Mexico on a holiday with her boy friend. She had some aversion to the use of the diaphragm, so her partner would insert it and take it out—a procedure he thoroughly enjoyed.

When their vacation came to an end, the young woman returned home and her lover returned to California, so she didn't see him for a while. Then she began to have a terrible vaginal discharge. She went to several physicians, who did not examine her but treated her with various types of douches, and the discharge continued to the point where she developed an irritation of her vulva and some odor.

When I examined her, the diaphragm was sitting high up in the vagina. It had been displaced and no longer covered the cervix, enabling her to menstruate without any difficulty. When I removed the diaphragm, she was terribly embarrassed, but she told me the entire story. She thought her partner had removed the diaphragm the last night they were in Mexico City. Apparently he had drunk too much tequila and forgotten.

Are there any side effects that may occur with the diaphragm?

There are some women who are allergic to certain jellies, so various types must be tried until we find one that causes no problem.

How long will a diaphragm last?

A considerable period of time—more than two years—if it is properly cared for. That means it must be washed, dried, and powdered after each use. However, as soon as the resiliency is lost or if there is the slightest question that the diaphragm won't stretch well, it's perfectly simple to buy another in the drugstore. All a woman needs to know is her size.

How do you account for the pregnancies which do seem to occur in women using the diaphragm?

Occasionally we run into a patient who has had not one, but two, pregnancies with the diaphragm, and we tend to feel that she is not using her diaphragm properly. Either she is not using it every single time from the very beginning of intercourse, or she is not using jelly, or she is not checking to be sure that the cervix is covered by the rubber. The diaphragm is a superb method of contraception, but it does require careful use every single time there is intercourse. The diaphragm should not be used as an adjunct to the dangerous rhythm method.

The only person who ever became pregnant after I fitted her with a diaphragm was a woman who understood the use of her diaphragm thoroughly and used it successfully for approximately six or eight months before she suddenly became pregnant. Because I was keeping data on diaphragm failures so that I could write a paper and could give better patient instruction, I went through all the particular checkpoints. Yes, she used the diaphragm every time from the beginning of intercourse. Yes, she always used extra jelly if she had intercourse more than one time during the night. She did everything exactly right. So how did she become pregnant?

"Dr. Flowers, I think I know what happened," she said, finally.

"Every now and then I have this incredible, shaking orgasm. And one morning after such an experience, I was getting ready to take out the diaphragm and I found it sitting sideways in my vagina."

What happened to this woman is rare, but it does happen because the vagina dilates during intercourse. It is for this reason that a diaphragm should always be tight-fitting—so it will not be displaced by the orgasmic response. Here again, an adequate amount of jelly on the diaphragm will provide additional protection.

Let's talk now about the rhythm method.

I am probably the most antirhythm doctor there ever was because it doesn't matter whether the woman uses the calendar rhythm method, the temperature method, or any other, she is eventually likely to get pregnant. That is why whenever I see a Catholic patient, I try to talk her out of using rhythm.

Unfortunately, it's not just Catholics who use this system. It has permeated our whole society, and many young people who are non-Catholics erroneously believe in it. But they should understand that the rhythm method is one of the two most common causes of pregnancy among patients who end up having abortions. The other common cause is the "bullet syndrome," in which the woman takes chances because she believes that pregnancy can never happen to her, just as soldiers during war take dangerous risks because they can't believe they will get shot.

But the rhythm method seems to make sense. If a woman refrains from intercourse around the time she is ovulating, how can she become pregnant?

The real problem with the rhythm method, even if it is used carefully and conscientiously, is that sperm can live in the woman's reproductive tract for four or five or maybe even seven days. A couple can have sex almost a week before any sign of ovulation, and that sex act can result in a pregnancy when ovulation finally occurs. The sperm just wait around, fully potent, until an egg is released.

The rhythm method can also fail if ovulation occurs later than usual, and the couple resumes having intercourse on the assumption that they are in a safe period.

I have collected data over a number of years on thoughtful, conscientious women who used extreme care with the rhythm method. Still they eventually became pregnant. This is why present data indicate that 14 to 15 women out of 100 using the rhythm method will become pregnant in a given year. And if the method is used haphazardly without proper understanding, as is so frequently done by the general population, the failure rate is about 35 percent. So rhythm is not something I can recommend.

What about the newer techniques of rhythm which test the cervical mucus?

These newer techniques are called natural birth control. They attempt to identify the time of ovulation by examination of the cervical mucus and by measuring the amount of carbohydrate. The mucus at the time of ovulation will look thin and rubbery and the sugar content will be elevated. The problem, of course, is that these signs of ovulation may come too late. The sperm from a previous intercourse may already be waiting inside the uterus or fallopian tubes.

Nevertheless, rhythm as a method of contraception is better than nothing, and if it's carried out carefully, if the cervical mucus is checked, and if the woman refrains from coitus from about the eighth day of the menstrual cycle until the twentieth day, very few pregnancies will occur. This is an extremely unsatisfactory method of contraception because it requires abstinence for at least twelve days at a time.

Why does the withdrawal method have so many failures? If a man removes his penis from the vagina before ejaculation, how can pregnancy result?

Pregnancy can occur because a man often loses his most potent sperm before he experiences the sensation of ejaculation. He can be totally unaware that he is impregnating the woman, or he may simply lose control and not be able to help it.

A young man once came to see me with his pregnant girl friend, who was a university student. He wanted to have a test done to determine if he was the father of her child. He was quite indignant, but the woman's story was straightforward. She told it with such ardor that I believed her when she said she had never had intercourse with anyone else. This fellow was absolutely sure, however, that the baby could not be his because he had never ejaculated in the woman's vagina. He had always practiced withdrawal.

He was amazed when I told him that withdrawal, or coitus interruptus, as it is otherwise known, is associated with a fairly high pregnancy rate and that men do in fact lose some sperm prior to the sensation of ejaculation.

What should a woman know about contraceptive foams and jellies?

Contraceptive foams and jellies are intended to kill sperm and are deposited with a plunger-type applicator up inside the vagina near the entrance to the uterus.

I feel that foam, if used without another contraceptive device such as a diaphragm or condom, is an unacceptable method of contraception simply because too many of my patients become pregnant using it. Foam dissipates in the vagina and doesn't form a sufficiently protective pool at the cervical entrance. Even when it's used conscientiously, the pregnancy rate is 5 to 10 percent, and that is just too high when there are more reliable methods available. Nor do I recommend the new foaming contraceptive vaginal tablets since they contain the same medical ingredient and work on the same principle as the vaginal foam.

Contraceptive jellies, on the other hand, have about half the pregnancy rate of foam—at least in my experience. So if a woman uses jelly very carefully and conscientiously, and does not play safe periods, the likelihood of a pregnancy is relatively small compared to the use of rhythm. Of course, if the jelly is used in conjunction with a diaphragm or condom, the pregnancy rate is even lower.

It should be noted, however, that jellies and foam can sometimes cause irritation or allergic reactions to the woman herself and to her partner.

Is douching an adequate method of contraception?

No, it is not, because the sperm travel up into the cervix in a matter of seven to ten seconds after the ejaculation of the male. By the time the woman gets out of bed, goes to the bathroom, and begins to wash out her vagina, it's already too late.

Douching is not only ineffective, it's a very unsatisfying method of contraception. The moments following coitus should be a time for pillow talk and a continuation of the warmth of lovemaking. It should not be necessary for the woman to jump out of a warm bed in the middle of the night to flush out her vagina—especially since it doesn't do much good anyway.

Is it possible for a woman to become pregnant without having an orgasm?

Indeed it is! Although the orgasmic response probably does increase fertility somewhat, because the contractions help move the sperm up through the vaginal canal, it is not necessary for a woman to have an orgasm in order to conceive.

What new contraceptives are now being developed?

Several new diaphragms are on the way. One is disposable while another is a small spongelike device which requires no jelly or cream and can be left in place one full month.

A vaginal ring is also being developed which slowly releases small amounts of progestin and can be kept in the vagina for a period of three months.

At the University of Alabama, we are developing a contraceptive called the micro-capsule which is inserted into the vagina. This gelatin capsule, which is smaller than the usual cold capsule, contains little particles of progestin or progesterone which move up into the uterus, where they coat the lining and prevent implantation. Our present studies indicate that these capsules should be inserted once a month.

We are also working to develop an injection that will act as a contraceptive for up to twelve months. This injection has advantages in addition to its mere convenience. It does not have to pass through the liver as do the oral contraceptives, and it provides a continuous but much smaller dose of hormones than the pill.

How are we coming along with the development of the male pill?

Unfortunately the male pill is still not working. The problem seems to be that as we reduce the production of sperm, we also reduce the man's sex drive. Attempts are being made to correct this problem by combining testosterone, the male hormone, with a substance that prevents the development of sperm. But we are using two very potent hormones, and the safety of this procedure has not yet been worked out.

Nevertheless, we are working on the problem, with the federal government and industry both spending millions and millions of dollars on this research. Women must not think they are being discriminated against in this regard.

6
PREGNANCY

If a man and woman are planning to have a child, what can they do before conception to ensure a normal, healthy baby?

I sincerely believe that a man and woman should go into training to have a child, just as an athlete goes into a period of training before he participates in a sporting event. I think it is most important that the couple be in good mental and physical health.

Hopefully they are not too obese, they have been eating properly, sleeping well and have not had a viral or infectious disease for six weeks before they attempt impregnation. If sickness does occur, the couple should stop trying for a conception and should use a birth control method until they have had a chance to recuperate fully. Many problems can arise if either partner is not in peak form. A viral infection may adversely affect a man's sperm, and he might produce a child with congenital abnormalities. Or a woman who has been ill may have inadequate development of the lining of the uterus, making implantation defective. So both partners should be in good physical condition and not have been sick for a period of six to eight weeks before pregnancy occurs.

Equally important is good psychological health. Men who are under tension tend to have lower sperm counts, and more abnormal sperm. Women who are under tension are more likely to have problems with the balance between their estrogen and progesterone, greater troubles with implantation, and possibly a greater chance of bearing children with birth defects. So if a husband and wife are living under excessive tension, if they are angry with each other for some reason, this is not a good time to attempt pregnancy.

What is the best intercourse position to promote conception?

I think that all gynecologists would agree that the preferable position is eyeball to eyeball in the "missionary position." It is also a good idea for the woman to have a pillow under her hips. After the man's ejaculation, the woman should pull up both of her knees and wrap her arms around them so that the cervix is actually sitting in a seminal pool. This is the position that is recommended for patients who have infertility problems, but I must assure you that conception can take place under all sorts of conditions and in all sorts of positions.

There are many reported cases where pregnancy has resulted from dry intercourse where an ejaculation occurred outside a vagina that was covered by underclothes. The sperm penetrated the material, passed through the vaginal secretions and moved on to the cervix— very rapidly.

Does frequent intercourse increase the likelihood of having a child?

Coitus four times a week is probably ideal. It is a mistake for couples to have intercourse less frequently in the hope of increasing their fertility. Infrequent intercourse may increase the total sperm count but not the number of effective sperm that may cause conception.

What are the earliest, most reliable tests for pregnancy?

The most reliable test, called the beta subunit test, measures a substance produced by the young embryo. This is a very sensitive test that can determine a pregnancy as early as two days before the missed menstrual period. This blood test requires sophisticated equipment and may not always be available in a smaller hospital setting, but the test is extremely accurate and dependable.

Three weeks after the first missed menstrual period, the more commonly used pregnancy test can be performed on the urine.

How accurate are the new "do-it-yourself" pregnancy tests?

These urine tests are much less reliable and may have a 10 to 15 percent error. They test for the presence of a substance known as human chorionic gonadotrophin (HCG), which is produced by the placenta.

What about false alarms? Are there ways to tell if a woman is not pregnant even if she has missed a menstrual period?

Although the earliest sign of pregnancy is a missed menstrual period, this symptom alone is not a 100 percent guarantee. A woman may have an occasional illness or emotional upset which changes her menstrual rhythm, or still more confusing, she may be *chronically* plagued with irregular periods. So if her breasts are not sore or tender, if she doesn't have a slight fullness in her face or a little bit of nausea, a woman can be reasonably sure she is not pregnant. Of course, if she has missed her period by two weeks or more, she can have a pregnancy test, which will usually give her a definite answer.

With contraception as reliable as it is today, are most pregnancies now planned?

The planning of pregnancy is related to socioeconomic group. Women in the upper groups have 80 percent of their pregnancies planned and wanted. Among patients in the lower groups, about 80 percent of the pregnancies are unplanned and probably unwanted. Among teenagers below the age of eighteen, over 90 percent of the pregnancies are unplanned and probably unwanted.

Once pregnancy occurs, how can a woman protect her unborn baby?

The most critical period of the baby's development is the first eight weeks of pregnancy, when the growing embryo begins to develop its heart, lungs, liver, and various other organs. Because certain infections can interfere with this process, a pregnant woman should do the best she can to avoid risk of viral infection. She should be around young children as little as possible because they are frequent carriers of infectious particles. During this first eight-week period she should stay out of crowds, and she should really try to protect herself from viral infections, such as mumps, measles, whooping cough, etc. This is extremely important because of the large number of birth defects— such as cataracts, heart and limb defects, as well as mental and sensory disorders—which are associated with early viral infections in the pregnant mother. Indeed, generalized viral infections are some of the major causes of cerebral palsy and mental retardation of the child. Mothers should also avoid contact with cats that hunt portions of their food, since they may carry toxoplasmosis, a cause of central nervous system damage.

The pregnant woman should also try to avoid all kinds of noxious materials, such as pesticides, and she should inform her obstetrician if she is taking any medication whatsoever, even aspirin. She should avoid cigarettes because we are finding that smoking seems to affect the fetus much more than we realized. It may retard the baby's growth, and it may have other subtle effects of which we are not aware. For those women who can't break the smoking habit, we ask that they cut down as much as possible.

That brings us to the matter of alcohol. Here, too, common sense is in order. The Food and Drug Administration recommends that pregnant woman not take more than two drinks a day, but I feel even this is too much. This is not meant to frighten a woman who drinks occasionally. But if a pregnant woman consumes large amounts of alcohol, the baby might be born with fetal alcohol syndrome, in which there are structural abnormalities and mental retardation. In these sad cases, the alcohol has affected the uterus and placenta, causing environmental problems for the baby in the womb.

Of course, most women are aware of the importance of good obstetrical care and of maintaining a well-balanced diet and avoiding emotional tension. Psychic stress can reduce blood flow to the uterus and, under extreme conditions, can damage the baby.

How should a woman go about selecting an obstetrician?

It is extremely important that every pregnant woman be under the care of a competent obstetrical team so that she can be checked regularly and can receive adequate advice concerning the progress of her pregnancy.

Aside from making certain that the obstetrician has been well trained and has had adequate experience, a woman must feel her physician is someone with whom she can communicate freely. There must be a feeling of rapport between them and a sense of working together as a team.

The day is gone, thank God, when the obstetrician made all the decisions and "took care of everything." It is the woman's body which produces and delivers the baby, and today's obstetrician functions as a captain and adviser, guiding the pregnancy ship through the channel and keeping it off the sandbars.

A woman should attempt to make certain that her obstetrician will be with her during the majority of labor, and she should express this expectation when she first meets with her physician. She should also let her preference be known concerning pain-killers (analgesia) and anesthesia, and she should determine her obstetrician's practices in this matter. If a woman really prefers natural childbirth, she should make certain her obstetrician will honor her wishes. And if she wants her husband to be with her during labor and delivery, she should make certain this is also agreeable to the physician.

Finally, the woman should be certain that her obstetrician is associated with a hospital that has a good reputation. The hospital should have a well-equipped and properly staffed nursery and preferably perform at least a thousand deliveries each year.

What can the obstetrician do to help the woman who has mixed or negative feelings about her pregnancy?

Probably the most helpful thing he can do is let her talk about her feelings. It is not up to the physician to try to convince a woman that she must adjust to the situation or accept her pregnancy if she has strong negative feelings. He should merely point out her options, which are to end the pregnancy, to have the baby and put it up for adoption, or to have the baby and keep it herself.

Of course, other problems may arise during this decision-making process. A patient may really want to terminate the pregnancy but have strong religious convictions which would prohibit an abortion. Then I would suggest that she see a clerical counselor.

Occasionally a patient's partner may be the one with mixed feelings because he is concerned about the financial responsibility. In situations of this type it is important to talk things out, preferably with both partners. The physician must be a patient listener; then it is his responsibility to spell out the options. But the decision must always be made by the patient.

Unfortunately, that was not the way it was in a recent case involving a pregnant young patient who came to me with several large masses in her abdomen. It was necessary to perform exploratory surgery to find out if these masses were fibroid tumors or possibly ovarian cancer. The patient was upset about her pregnancy and really wanted me to go ahead and perform a hysterectomy, removing the uterus, contents and all.

Her family, however, was very concerned. Her father, mother, and aunt all came to the hospital when we were discussing the pros and cons of this problem, and although the patient was unmarried, her relatives really wanted her to have this baby.

I explained to the patient that her family should have nothing to say about this matter. This was her pregnancy, and the decision was up to her.

She finally decided to follow her family's wishes. I operated on her and found fibroids that were tremendous in size, almost filling the entire abdomen. Since we had ruled out cancer, I closed the abdomen and kept a careful watch over this young woman for the rest of her pregnancy. She didn't smile very much during this time. She had tremendous discomfort and pain, but she did have her baby. And when she left the hospital, members of her family took turns carrying her infant.

Now that "preparation for childbirth" is very much in vogue, could you explain what goes on in this process?

Preparation for childbirth is simply a method of making certain that a woman is prepared, both physically and emotionally, for childbirth. Although she will be trained in the principles of *natural* childbirth, that does not mean that she may not require some pain relief during labor and delivery. It only means that she will be taught how to breathe, how to relax, and how to understand what is happening in her body. She will learn exactly what is happening in the growth and development of the fetus. She will be told what is going to happen during labor, who is going to be with her, and what she is supposed to do. She will be taught how to position herself in labor, how to push down, and how to birth a baby, which in many ways is an athletic activity involving coordination of many muscles. She will be taught how to strain down on the voluntary muscles while the muscles of the uterus contract involuntarily. Women who have all this information are much less afraid of the perfectly normal, natural process of labor and delivery.

Another advantage of this type of training is that it improves the doctor-patient relationship. When I deliver a baby, I feel like a coach at an athletic event, and I want the woman to know how to play the game.

From her point of view, preparation for childbirth often builds confidence in the obstetrician. She learns to trust that the doctor will call the right plays at the right time and will correct the plays if things are not going well.

Preparation for childbirth also involves the husband, and this gives the woman a cheering section. A thoughtful, motivated, affectionate husband who has gone through the same lectures on preparation for childbirth can help his wife learn how to breathe, how to relax, how to push down. I feel very strongly that unless there are unusual circumstances, it's great for the husband to be with his wife during labor and delivery. And he should be more than a curious bystander. He should be there to give support and helpful encouragement and to share in this extremely important occasion in both their lives.

What are the most common fears you encounter concerning pregnancy?

Probably the most terrifying fear of all involves having an abnormal child. Fortunately we can now test for a number of abnormalities long before birth so that parents can have the option of aborting an abnormal baby. There is no way, however, to test for every conceivable problem, and there is no guarantee of a healthy child. So this can be a very worrisome thing to some women, especially those who have had problems before.

Other people are concerned about losing their independence and about the sheer responsibility of raising a child. Still others may worry how the arrival of a baby will interfere with the parents' relationship.

These are all very important points for the couple to discuss and work out with the assistance of their physician if necessary.

I discovered long ago that one way to uncover hidden fears about pregnancy is to ask pregnant women to tell me about their dreams. Women themselves should initiate this type of discussion if they find they are having unusual dreams so that they can discuss them and develop some insight into their true feelings. Sometimes these dreams are veiled in absurdities, but the major feeling is often there, and dreams are extremely important in determining what fears are present.

I have had pregnant women tell me they dreamed of a dog with only three legs or some type of grotesque figure, indicating that they were fearful of having an abnormal child.

Occasionally a woman will fear losing her figure. I have had reports of dreams where the woman's legs became extremely fat and flesh actually hung over her ankles. The woman who has this type of fear may be insecure in herself and in her marriage.

You haven't mentioned fear of labor and delivery.

This fear is not nearly as great as it used to be. While there is still some dread of labor, most women today realize that having a baby is not the life-threatening process it once was.

Of course, the patient's attitude toward labor is formed by her own background. If her mother spoke of childbirth as an experience of suffering, the daughter will probably acquire a certain amount of anxiety of her own. This anxiety will affect her choice of delivery technique, her choice of anesthesia and even her choice of a physician.

Fear of labor and delivery can actually prolong and complicate the process. Fear will cause the woman to produce adrenaline, which is nature's way of preparing her for a dangerous situation. But adrenaline will slow down uterine contractions—or, worse yet, cause them to cease entirely. So it is important that fear be kept to a minimum—especially fear of the unknown. And that is why education in childbirth is so essential. It has been my experience that by explaining to the woman exactly what will happen during labor and delivery and by assuring her that she will not be alone, we avoid unnecessary anesthesia and many kinds of obstetric complications.

Many women today remain active during pregnancy. Is this a healthy trend?

While I encourage women to keep themselves involved in interesting activities, pregnancy is a time when extra demands are being made upon the body, and periods of rest are extremely important.

Remember that the body is concentrating on allowing this fetus to grow, and this growth requires that the fetus be adequately nourished by uterine blood flow. If a woman walks around and expends extra energy, her blood will first supply her muscles, which have top priority. This is a throwback to earlier times when it was most important for a person to be able to defend himself or herself against any predator.

But pregnant women should keep in mind that excessive and tiring work or exercise are not good for the baby. So rest is important during pregnancy, particularly for women who have heart trouble, high blood pressure, or kidney or liver disease. That means a rest period in both the morning and the afternoon, for when a woman rests, she is allowing maximum blood flow to the uterus. Incidentally, it is better for her to rest on her left side, because then the uterus is not causing pressure on the great vessels that lead to the heart. Of course, bedtime should also be at a reasonable hour.

How do you feel about women working during pregnancy?

I personally feel a woman should not work after the twenty-eighth week of pregnancy. If she does work, it should probably be only half time. During the final trimester of pregnancy, the heart is working 35 percent harder than normal, and this is not something to be taken lightly. That is why I feel a pregnant woman should lead a fairly relaxed life and not become fatigued.

There is still much confusion about how much weight a woman should gain during pregnancy.

Unfortunately there are still many obstetricians who feel that weight gain should be restricted during pregnancy. That philosophy started years ago when some data were published indicating that women who gained over thirty pounds were more likely to develop hypertension (or toxemia, as it was called in those days). Now it *is* true that women who gain excessive amounts of fluid are more prone to high blood pressure. But that occurs only when the weight gain is comprised of fluid. So if a woman gains twenty-five to thirty-five pounds during pregnancy, that is in no way detrimental; in fact, it is to be desired as long as she is not troubled by swelling of the hands and face. Some swelling of the feet is normal.

Moreover, if we are dealing with a woman who is overweight to begin with, it would be most unrealistic, and even undesirable, for this patient not to gain at least twenty-five to thirty pounds during pregnancy. Despite those physicians who unfortunately believe that women who are overweight should diet during pregnancy, this is just not the time to go on a diet.

How much exercise is permissible?

Only that amount which does not cause fatigue. Somewhere along the way women began thinking that it was a good idea for them to walk a mile each day when they were pregnant. This idea developed in European countries where people are more athletic in general and where more emphasis is placed on exercise as preparation for childbirth. If a woman wants to carry out this regimen while she is pregnant, that's fine—as long as she has her physician's approval. It's always a good thing to maintain good muscle tone, but this exercise will have very little to do with labor and delivery. There is nothing about childbearing that demands an athletic degree of muscle coordination and strength. Labor is not like playing tennis or lifting weights or running a marathon. You are going to birth a child, and the birthing of this child is primarily done through involuntary contractions of the uterus, which is a smooth muscle that all the exercise in the world is not going to affect.

So a pregnant woman who is engaged in all the physical activities of caring for a home and a family must not feel that she should walk a mile at the end of each day. It is much more important that she not become unduly fatigued.

Could you describe how the baby develops during the nine months of pregnancy?

After conception occurs in the fallopian tube, the fertilized egg travels through the tube and reaches the uterus in approximately three days. It floats freely within the uterus for an additional three days and then imbeds itself in the lining of the uterus. After this implantation, the product of conception divides itself into two parts: the embryo and the placenta. The placenta in mammals is similar to the roots of a tree. It consists of multiple branching tubes that extract from the mother all of the oxygen, vitamins, minerals and food nutrients needed by the developing fetus. It also sends back to the mother all of the waste products of the fetus. If all of its branches were flattened, the placenta would, at the time of birth, have the surface area of a ten-by-twelve-foot rug, but it is actually compacted into a small disc measuring seven inches in diameter and weighing one pound.

The embryo has completely formed all of its organs and extremities by the eighth week of life. Thus all congenital abnormalities will have occurred by that time. This is why it is so important to avoid viral infections and noxious substances during the early weeks of pregnancy.

When the fetus is four months old, it weighs approximately three ounces. When it is six months old, it weighs about twenty ounces. At eight months its weight is around three pounds, and the average weight at birth is six and a half to seven and a half pounds.

What are the most common complications of pregnancy?

Topping the list is hypertension, and this problem often arises during the second or third trimester if the body does not adjust to the extra workload being placed upon it. The treatment for this problem is bed rest, bed rest, and more bed rest. Because hypertension causes the blood vessels to become constricted (more narrow), the blood flow to the uterus is reduced. So the patient must rest to ensure adequate blood supply and appropriate nourishment for the fetus. The same thing is true when a pregnant woman has heart or kidney disease.

Diabetes is another major complication of pregnancy which is becoming more and more frequent. That is because our treatment for diabetes has improved, and more diabetics are able to become pregnant. In this case, it is extremely important to keep strict control of the blood-sugar levels with the use of insulin. This requires an extremely motivated, intelligent patient who will follow a diet very carefully down to the last ten or fifteen calories a day. Such a patient must also take the prescribed insulin very carefully and come to see her doctor at frequent intervals, so he can be sure that the regulation is correct. The regimen for a pregnant diabetic also involves bed rest and restriction of physical activity. But more than anything else, it involves intelligent cooperation.

Still another major complication of pregnancy is kidney infection. During pregnancy, the renal system does not work as well as it does in a nonpregnant state. This is because the kidneys, ureters, and bladder lose some of their muscle tone and the urine does not flow as well.

This is one of the reasons that pregnant women seem more subject to urinary-tract infections. The other reason is that the woman's natural immunity is reduced during pregnancy, possibly in order to prevent rejection of the embryo. We must remember that the embryo is really a foreign body inside the mother, and her immune responses would normally try to reject this alien material. So nature turns the immune system down, but this creates other problems. The ability of the body to resist the infection is greatly impaired, and all types of infections, be they pneumonia, liver disease, or urinary-tract infections, are more serious in the pregnant woman. They last longer and are harder to treat.

Even worse, some urinary-tract infections may affect the uterus and cause premature labor and delivery—at a time before the baby is equipped to survive outside the womb. This happens because the kidneys and uterus are formed from similar embryonic tissue, so when infection causes irritation and contractions in the kidney, the uterus begins to contract as well, and the premature onset of labor occurs. If this happens, a woman should contact her obstetrician immediately because there are drugs which are often successful in stopping such labor.

It's important for pregnant women who have kidney infection to obtain adequate rest, to drink plenty of water so they can keep their kidneys flushed, and to have regular cultures of their urine taken so that an antibiotic can be prescribed if they have a severe problem. If there should be an onset of labor pains, they should immediately report to the hospital so they can receive the proper medications to stop the labor.

One more thing: it is recommended that any woman who has any of the more serious conditions we have discussed—heart disease, hypertension, diabetes, or kidney disease—receive her obstetrical care in a special "high-risk program." In such a program, a team of specialists will collaborate on the complexities of her problem and will be much better able to prevent and handle obstetrical emergencies should they arise.

You haven't mentioned one problem I've often heard about—the Rh problem.

This problem arises when the mother with Rh-negative blood gives birth to a baby who is Rh-positive. During the delivery process some of the baby's blood enters the mother's bloodstream and she develops antibodies to any future Rh-positive babies which may be conceived. In subsequent pregnancies, these Rh antibodies from the mother's blood will cross the placenta and damage the new baby's blood cells, making it anemic. Occasionally it is necessary to transfuse the baby inside the uterus or to induce early delivery if the baby begins to have serious impairment.

The Rh problem has essentially been conquered today by giving every Rh-negative woman who aborts or delivers a full-term or premature infant a substance which destroys the baby's Rh-positive red cells. This prevents the mother from developing an allergic response to any future Rh-positive babies. Every Rh-negative mother should insist that she receive this drug, called RhoGam, following a delivery, abortion, or miscarriage.

What is meant by placenta previa?

This problem occurs when the placenta grows in the lower rather than the upper part of the womb and becomes detached from the uterine wall, causing bleeding. This serious problem, the likelihood of which increases with age, number of children, and inadequate blood supply to the uterus, sometimes requires that the baby be delivered prematurely. Anytime a woman has bleeding during pregnancy, she must contact her physician immediately or go to a hospital where appropriate tests can be carried out to make the critical decision of what to do about the baby.

Today we use sonar—the same system that the navy uses to detect submarines—to accurately locate the placenta in the womb. Therefore our diagnosis is very accurate, and the condition can be treated appropriately.

We now try to take a more conservative approach to the treatment of placenta previa. We sometimes send the patient home after the bleeding stops so that the fetus can have more time to grow in the uterus. But the cooperation of the mother is of tremendous importance. First, she must not have intercourse. She must rest. She must not work. She must not exert herself, and she must never go anywhere without a companion who could bring her back to the hospital immediately if she has a repeat hemorrhage.

Another type of placental separation sometimes occurs just prior to delivery, and this is a more serious complication, known as premature separation of the placenta. It is frequently accompanied by elevation in blood pressure and can be very dangerous to both the mother and baby. The symptoms here are severe abdominal pain and bleeding. These symptoms should always alert the patient to a major problem.

Is it permissible for a pregnant woman to have intercourse?

Absolutely. If she is in good health, there is no reason why a woman should not have intercourse throughout her entire pregnancy right up till the time she goes into labor. The notion that intercourse during the first three months of pregnancy causes miscarriage was perpetuated years ago when it was not realized that the majority of miscarriages are caused by chromosomal defects in the embryo. Such miscarriages are nature's way of ending a pregnancy because there is some abnormality in the baby, and this problem has nothing to do with intercourse during pregnancy.

Now the other old wives' tale—that a woman should not have intercourse during the final six weeks of pregnancy—grew out of the belief that intercourse might cause infection or premature rupture of the membranes. Again this has been proven incorrect. We have found that women who have intercourse up to the very end of pregnancy have no more problems with infection or ruptured membranes than women who are abstaining.

One can see how both of these myths got started. Women who were having intercourse during the first three months occasionally had a spontaneous abortion. And women who had intercourse during the last six weeks of pregnancy occasionally had premature rupture of the membranes. We now have good studies which indicate that intercourse was not to blame in either of these cases, but there remains the old puritanical belief that there is something sinful or dirty about a pregnant woman's having sex.

Why do some women seem to have less sexual appetite when they are pregnant?

A woman should understand that during the first three months of pregnancy she may feel an aversion to sexual intercourse. This reduction in sexual appetite may be the result of hormonal adjustments during this period, or it may be due to the woman's belief that intercourse may cause harm to the fetus or even cause miscarriage.

It is interesting to note that the human primate is the only animal that continues to have intercourse during pregnancy. All other primates—the great apes, baboons, and monkeys—cease coitus during this time, possibly because nature may have decided that a sex drive is needed only during those periods when the female could become pregnant.

So this reduction in sex drive during pregnancy has been present for millions of years, and this hasn't changed much in lower animals.

Something has changed, however, with regard to human sexuality, and it is possibly related to the growth of the human brain, which has almost doubled in size. It's quite conceivable that with the development of the thinking portion of the brain, or frontal lobes as they are called, the human female developed the need for affection.

It has also been during the last half million years that families have developed, and this too would foster coitus during pregnancy. The woman would want to please her husband, and his physical desires would be present she was pregnant or not.

On the other hand, some pregnant women feel sexier than ever. This drive is probably psychological, not hormonal, in nature. It is probably related to the woman's desire to be loved and protected during this period when she feels more insecure and vulnerable. Love-making is a way to give and receive affection at a time when a woman may not be quite as sure of herself and of her own physical attractiveness.

I recall one patient for whom this became a problem. She came to see me when she was about thirty-six weeks pregnant, and she had tears running down her cheeks as she walked in and closed my office door. "Dr. Flowers," she said, "I just can't stand it any longer."

"Well, let's talk about what you can't stand," I replied. "What is the problem?"

"My husband won't make love to me," she explained. "During the last month he has had no interest in me, and when I make advances to him, he kind of puts me off and says, 'You know we shouldn't be doing this sort of thing right now.'

"I told him that you assured me it was perfectly all right to make love during pregnancy. I am dreaming about it at night and getting more and more upset."

I knew this woman's husband, so I called him soon after she left my office. I asked him to come down to the office because this was not something I could discuss over the phone.

I found there was no other woman in his life, and there was good affection between him and his wife. The real problem was that his wife's being pregnant turned him off. There were several events in his childhood that probably accounted for this.

When this man was about twelve or thirteen years old, his mother became pregnant with his younger brother. One day the mother slipped and fell and had to spend some time in the hospital. When she finally returned home everybody treated her with such extreme care that he began to think of a pregnant woman as something very, very fragile. A discussion of how he had developed this attitude allowed him to gradually initiate coitus, and his wife was reassured.

Is orgasm harmful to the fetus?

Not in any way. Orgasm does cause some uterine contractions, but unless those contractions are multiple over a period of time, they do not trip the mechanism of labor. And to deny a woman something as natural and spontaneous as intercourse and orgasm may well have greater consequences.

Can the pressure of a man's body on the abdomen be harmful to the fetus?

The fetus is insulated with amniotic fluid, so this is really no problem, although some women might find it more comfortable to assume the female-superior, or upper straddling, position. Other couples find the entry of the vagina from the rear more satisfactory, while still others prefer intercourse on the side. If the rear-entry position is used, it may be helpful for the woman to apply pressure on a small pillow placed directly against the clitoris so there will be stimulation to achieve orgasm.

Why does the pregnant belly feel so hard to the touch?

Actually it doesn't feel hard to the knowledgeable examiner. An experienced obstetrician can tell when he's feeling the buttocks or the head of the baby in the uterus. Sometimes the mother will feel the baby's buttocks, or his head or back, and this feels hard. But if she would feel a little bit over to the side, she would feel the soft uterus filled with amniotic fluid.

How early in the pregnancy can a doctor predict twins or triplets?

An obstetrician can usually begin to suspect multiple births around the sixteenth week of pregnancy if the uterus is larger than normal. If he wants to confirm his diagnosis, he can use sonar, which is a totally safe method. Sonar uses sound waves, which are bounced off the fetus floating in its amniotic fluid.

Why do multiple births sometimes come as a surprise?

A physician will rarely miss multiple births today if he is checking the growth of the abdomen and using sonar—and later X ray—if he suspects twins. He may, however, not be able to tell if triplets or quadruplets are arriving because it is difficult to be sure of the exact number of babies when there are so many fetuses involved.

It is extremely important, however, for the physician to know when there will be multiple births. Often a cesarean section is required, so these cases should not come as a surprise if a woman has had proper prenatal care.

Of course, if a woman just shows up in active labor and this is the first chance the obstetrician has had to examine her, it is sometimes difficult to pick up two fetal heartbeats and difficult to feel two babies.

I received a good lesson in this problem when I was a medical student at Johns Hopkins thirty-five years ago. We were allowed to deliver those women who had already borne a previous child, and the interns and residents generally delivered those women who were having their first baby or who were expected to have complications.

One day I was assigned a patient who had already had five children, but during this pregnancy she had never been to an obstetrician and she had not had prenatal care. She just walked into the hospital when she began labor.

To all appearances, she was having a very rapid labor. I began checking her progress and became a little suspicious that the head size of the baby was not as big as it should be for the size of the abdomen. But I was only a medical student; I hadn't been on obstetrics too long, and I really didn't have the courage to bring this up to the resident who was supervising me. So I kept it to myself.

When the time came for the baby to arrive, the resident was involved with an obstetric complication in the next delivery room, so I performed the delivery myself. The baby was born with no trouble, but when I put my hand upon the uterus to check on the placenta, it was perfectly clear that there was another baby still inside.

I immediately instructed the nurse to call the resident, but he was still unable to leave his patient. He had one of the other residents paged, but before that resident could arrive, the second baby was born. Again I reached up to check on the placenta, and again it was obvious there was still another baby. And that's how I became the only medical student at Johns Hopkins ever to deliver triplets. I can assure you that the chief resident would have loved to deliver those babies, but he never had a chance.

Could we talk for a moment about teenage pregnancy? Why is this considered a high-risk problem?

I personally feel that pregnancies that occur before the age of eighteen are biological mistakes. This would be particularly true of pregnancies in girls around the age of eleven or twelve.

I say this first because young girls were not meant to menstruate as early as they now do. In the mid-1800s the average age of onset of menstruation was sixteen. Now the average age is eleven.

This means that young girls today are activating the sexual centers of their brain at an earlier and earlier age. Apparently this change is caused by the fact that we are feeding our children better than ever and are causing them to grow more rapidly. The onset of menstruation is related to a certain body weight, about 105 pounds, and to a certain head size that allows the development of the hypothalamus, which produces the hormones that stimulate the ovaries.

A young girl below the age of eighteen is still growing—her bones are growing, her heart is developing, her liver is growing, her kidney and vascular systems are developing—then suddenly there is added to all this growth activity the additional burden of a pregnancy, which causes a 35 percent increase in the body's workload. So a number of complications are possible. The most common of these is high blood pressure, but teenagers also tend to have more difficult labors and deliveries because often their pelvis has not yet reached full growth.

And, of course, there are psychological problems. Many of these youngsters regret the pregnancy and often try to deny it to themselves to the point where they neglect their own care. When they do come for checkups and treatment, they make difficult patients. They don't abide by our advice. They eat improperly, rest improperly and generally ignore our instructions. Consequently, minor complications which could have been corrected become major. Their minor hypertension can get out of hand and lead to convulsions. A small amount of urinary-tract infection can lead to a severe renal infection that can damage their kidneys for the rest of their lives. A small amount of anemia can become a major problem. These are some of the reasons the teenage pregnancy is high risk.

A recent case I know of involved a girl who withheld the fact that she was pregnant from her family and friends and refused to have medical assistance. She bought tighter and tighter corsets and continued to go to school. She developed swelling of the face and began to gain weight. She went on a near-starvation diet in an effort to keep her weight within normal limits. Eventually, when she began to have severe headaches, she took large amounts of aspirin. She developed severe hypertension with constriction of her blood vessels and a reduction of the blood supply to all her vital organs, along with a reduction of blood supply to her fetus. This girl eventually convulsed, lost the fetus, and almost lost her life. Because her high blood pressure went unchecked, she suffered a stroke and today has a weakness in one of her legs.

What special care do you suggest for pregnant teenagers?

I have a general philosophy that an unmarried teenager should either have an abortion or receive some type of domiciliary care. This would mean that she would go to a special school where she would have at least two well-balanced meals provided each day. She would be encouraged to rest in the morning and afternoon, and she would have group psychotherapy so that she would understand the problems of her own self-image which led to the pregnancy in the first place. She should also receive advice on how to take care of her baby and how to use contraceptives in the future. She could continue her schooling, of course, and then go home to her own family at night.

In this way the girl and her baby would have the best chance for a good start on their new life.

What are the most common causes of miscarriage and premature births?

Fifty percent of all spontaneous abortions (or miscarriages) are caused by chromosome abnormalities. That is why a woman who miscarries repeatedly must have chromosomal studies performed to be sure she is not going to have an abnormal child in later pregnancies. She should also have studies of her uterus (uterosalpingogram or X-ray studies) and appropriate endocrine studies to determine if the lining of her uterus is favorable for an embryo to implant and grow. Over 90 percent of spontaneous abortions are due to abnormalities of the embryo, uterus, or uterine lining.

Today we can detect some sixty serious problems before birth, and if necessary and desired by the mother, we can terminate the pregnancy. Geneticists can also detect carriers of hereditary disease and can counsel them on their risk of having an abnormal child. So before any couple jumps to the conclusion that they have a hereditary problem, possibly because they have already had one abnormal child, they should seek the advice of a specialist. Many so-called birth defects, such as cerebral palsy, hydrocephalus, and sensory or hearing disorders, are not related to any problem with the genes but are caused by some injury at birth or some type of viral infection during pregnancy or soon after delivery. Parents of such children need special counseling about the risk of recurrence along with some reassurance that this particular problem is not of genetic origin. Often couples will deny themselves the privilege of having a normal, healthy baby because of an unfounded fear of having another handicapped child.

This brings to mind an attractive couple I once met at a cocktail party. As we were talking about the prospects of our local football team, the husband suddenly became very serious and said, "Dr. Flowers, we have a child with cerebral palsy, but my wife doesn't like to talk about it." They went ahead and recounted the story of the child who was partially deaf, could not see very well, and could only crawl. This problem was a tremendous burden on the wife, and she rarely left the house because she was frightened to leave the child with a babysitter.

It became apparent that the wife had a great guilt complex. She had frankly admitted to her husband that she had had intercourse before she was married, and she was afraid she was being punished for this "sin." They were quite an affectionate couple and really wanted to have another child but were scared to death. They had never really discussed this problem with a physician and had never gone back to the obstetrician who delivered their affected child.

I explained the complexities of the situation but told the couple that there are certain factors of cerebral palsy that are not genetic. There might be no reason at all to suspect that another child would be afflicted.

So I wrote to the obstetrician who had delivered the baby, and he replied that there was no question but that this child's cerebral palsy was due to an infection. The doctor was absolutely sure this infection was the cause of brain damage and the couple should have no hesitation about another pregnancy.

When I gave this information to the couple, they were extraordinarily pleased. They went ahead and had another child, who turned out to be perfectly normal. This case illustrates the importance of obtaining good data regarding so-called genetic problems.

I remember another couple who came in quite concerned about the fact that they had had a child with multiple abnormalities. The baby had died, but unfortunately, the parents were never told the exact nature of the abnormalities. I wrote to the obstetrician and the pediatrician but the child had never been X-rayed or diagnosed carefully, and an autopsy had not been done after the child died. So there was really no way to determine the types of defects involved or to know what the risk might be in having another child.

This problem illustrates how important it is when an infant dies of a serious defect that the couple be sure that an autopsy is performed, X rays taken, and chromosomal analysis made. These studies will, in general, give an accurate diagnosis of the cause and possible risk of recurrence of infants with similar abnormalities. For those couples who need more information on genetic problems, a good place to turn is the March of Dimes International Directory of Genetic Services.

What causes genetic disorders?

There are three main causes of genetic defects: single-gene defects (involving dominant, recessive, and sex-linked problems), chromosomal abnormalities, and a combination of other factors.

Let's deal first with single- or dominant-gene defects, where only one parent need be a carrier to pass the problem on to the child. If the male partner has Huntington's chorea, for instance, a disease which involves progressive deterioration of the brain, his children stand a fifty-fifty chance of inheriting the disease.

Recessive gene defects, on the other hand, require both parents to transmit the defect, as in Tay-Sachs disease, cystic fibrosis, or sickle-cell anemia. If only one parent contributes the recessive gene to the new baby, the child will become a carrier but will not have the disease.

Just about everybody carries a number of defective recessive genes, which are harmless in single doses. The problem appears only when two people with the same defective recessive gene reproduce. Then the odds are one in four that the offspring will be affected.

Next we come to sex-linked defects, or X-linked recessive disorders, which show up only in males, although they are carried by females. One classic example of this problem is hemophilia. Another is muscular dystrophy. Fortunately we can now usually detect female carriers of this disease in its most severe form. A new test is also being developed which involves the chemical study of cells taken from the amniotic fluid during pregnancy to determine if the fetus is affected.

I recall one pregnant patient who had had a previous child born with Duchenne's muscular dystrophy. This is a terrible disease which cripples the child and eventually kills him, often before adolescence. This woman was terribly frightened about having another child with this condition, and when she became pregnant she was almost psychotic with fear. She was extremely depressed and talked about suicide. We withdrew some cells from the amniotic fluid and determined that the fetus was a female. This, of course, was good news. It absolutely eliminated the possibility of this woman's having another child with Duchenne's muscular dystrophy, because females can be carriers but they cannot have the disease.

What happens with chromosome abnormalities?

Chromosomal abnormalities can lead to structural problems, such as an undersized head, a flat or moon-shaped face, a drooping eyelid, turned-down corners of the mouth, even failure to develop hands or feet.

There are a number of these abnormalities that can cause mental retardation, but the most common chromosome abnormality is Down's syndrome, or mongolism, which can be caused by an abnormal chromosome from the mother or father, or sometimes by a fertilization accident. Down's syndrome is related to maternal aging—that is, the older the woman is at the time of pregnancy, the higher the risk of the baby having Down's syndrome. The chances of a woman who is 25 years old producing a mongoloid child are about 1 in 1500. This risk increases to 1 in 300 for women at the age of 35. And for women who are 40, the risk is 1 in 40. That is why all pregnant women above the age of 35 should have amniocentesis to make certain their baby does not have Down's syndrome—if they are willing to consider termination of the pregnancy if the child is affected.

You have mentioned genetic disorders caused by a combination of factors. Could you say a little more about these?

These problems, known as "multifactorial" or "polygenetic" disorders, involve more than one defective gene, and they may result in a cleft lip, cleft palate, heart defect, dislocation of the hip, obstruction of the small bowel, and—most dreadful of all—abnormalities of the spinal column or brain. The general risk of having this type of defect is about 1 in 600, but if a woman has had one child with this problem, her risk increases to 1 in 20.

Fortunately today amniocentesis can give us some indication of whether a fetus is affected, and the parents can have the opportunity to terminate the pregnancy. The sonar technique is also being improved rapidly to the point where we are able to pick up more and more anatomical abnormalities. And still other techniques are being developed which will allow visualization of the fetus in utero and sampling of its blood.

What happens during amniocentesis?

This is an office procedure that is generally performed when a woman is approximately sixteen weeks pregnant. A small amount of local anesthesia is used, and there is minimal discomfort to the patient. Twenty or 30 cc of amniotic fluid are drawn out of the uterus with a sterile syringe. This material is gently handled and transferred to the genetic laboratory, taking care that the cells are not injured in any way. They are then placed in an appropriate broth and allowed to grow for ten to twenty-one days. What you finally do with these cells depends on what you are testing for. We may study the chromosomes or we may do chemical analysis of the cells to determine metabolic birth defects. But we are not able to test for all known disorders.

In addition to performing amniocentesis on women over the age of thirty-five, we recommend the procedure for women who have a family history of genetic disorders or who have had previous children with genetic problems.

Is amniocentesis dangerous?

Not if performed properly. In any invasive procedure, such as amniocentesis, a spinal tap, or looking at the bronchial tubes, there are always potential hazards. However, a collaborative study was performed by the National Institutes of Health which indicated there were no greater dangers to a fetus whose mother had an amniocentesis than to a fetus in a group of appropriately matched controls.

What advice can you give to couples who are unable to have a child?

First, I think it is important to define what we mean by infertility. If a couple have been unable to have a child even though they have been having intercourse at least two times each week for a period of one year, they may indeed have a problem.

Unfortunately, about fifteen out of every hundred married couples in this country are involuntarily childless, and these couples deserve a thorough examination because a large percentage can be helped.

We should realize, however, that there are certain aspects of fertility over which we have no control—for instance, age. We know that a woman is most fertile between the ages of eighteen and twenty-five; her fertility declines after the age of thirty or thirty-five. That is one reason we encourage women to have their pregnancies before they are thirty to thirty-five years old. They will not only have fewer miscarriages and other obstetrical problems, they will be able to conceive far more easily.

What about the man's ability to father a child? Does this decrease with age?

Yes. The male's fertility reaches its peak around the age of twenty-four or twenty-five and diminishes around the age of forty. Although he is certainly able to father a child late into life, this ability does decrease with advancing years.

It is important to note that fertility problems in the male account for about 30 percent of the childless couples we see. That is why it is extremely important, when fertility problems occur, that adequate diagnostic studies be performed on the male.

What are the major causes of infertility in women?

Abnormalities of the fallopian tubes account for 35 percent of fertility problems in women. The tubes may be underdeveloped or damaged by infection. Abnormalities of the cervix account for another 20 percent, and hormonal factors for about 25 percent. Infertility may also be caused by endometriosis, and occasionally we find a woman who is allergic to her husband's sperm.

Probably the next two most common causes of infertility in women are the inability to ovulate and failure to maintain the proper hormonal environment for the implanted embryo.

Can these problems be treated?

Sometimes they can. If the failure to ovulate is caused by obesity, chronic anxiety, heavy smoking, and drinking, the woman may be able to correct her problem by changing her habits and modifying her life-style. If this fails, however, we do have medication which will induce ovulation, but this can be expensive and should be used only under the close supervision of a fertility specialist. Improvement in the uterine lining's sugars and enzymes can be effected by giving progesterone hormone if there are problems with implantation.

If a woman has problems with her fallopian tubes, how successful is tubal surgery?

This form of surgery is only 10 to 15 percent successful if the obstruction is due to pelvic infection. However, it is successful 30 to 60 percent of the time if the obstruction is due to a previously performed tubal ligation for sterilization in the female. We are very successful in reversing sterilization, but tubal surgery should only be performed by a surgeon who specializes in this technique. He must use the very latest techniques of magnification and very small sutures. The first attempt at reanastomosis (or reuniting the tubes) is the most likely one to succeed.

What types of problems can cause a man to be sterile?

The obvious ones are overweight, fatigue, excessive smoking or drinking, diabetes, plus all the other psychological factors which may interfere with his having coitus. He may have certain developmental problems, such as undescended testes, abnormalities of the penis, or enlarged veins in his scrotum. He may have hormonal problems, such as thyroid disease or a failure of the pituitary hypothalamus to stimulate the testes to produce sperm. He may have had mumps or other viral infections. He may have had gonorrhea, which can inflame the testicles, or he may have an inflammation of the prostate, which may or may not be related to previous venereal disease. So you see there are many possible causes of infertility in men.

There may also be environmental problems. One of these is heat around the scrotum. A truck driver, taxi driver, or any other man who sits for long periods of time in heated areas so that his scrotum remains close to his body may not produce enough sperm. Of course, previous exposure to radiation or toxic substances can also cause problems.

All these things are important, so whenever there is a problem of infertility, certain tests should be performed on the man. He should have a careful examination, including the penis and scrotum. He should have a thyroid test and a prostate test and his semen should be examined for the appearance of the sperm and the presence or absence of infection. But it is not necessary to abstain from coitus prior to the sperm count, which is performed from a masturbation specimen.

What if the physician can find no reason for the infertility?

This is our most difficult problem. If a thorough examination with all the necessary tests does not uncover a cause of infertility in either partner, it may be that there are psychological factors. Or it may be that we just don't have enough information at the present time to help this particular couple. I never tell a couple that pregnancy absolutely cannot occur unless I believe it is really impossible. Occasionally a pregnancy will occur in these cases, and the couple feels much happier having some hope. It is also important for the woman to continue to consult her gynecologist at six-to-twelve-month intervals to be sure situations have not changed or medications become available which may be of help.

When do you recommend artificial insemination?

If the problems of infertility originate with the husband, and if these problems are uncorrectible, we can now offer artificial insemination with the sperm of a volunteer donor.

This is a controversial technique, but it can be done quite successfully if a couple is certain that they want to have a child in this manner.

The laws regarding artificial insemination vary from state to state.

In some places the husband must actually adopt the child, but in other states it is necessary only for him to sign the birth certificate.

How are donors selected?

We try to pick a healthy donor who has previously fathered a healthy child. We obtain the donor's genetic history as best we can, and we try to pick a donor who resembles the husband in appearance as much as possible. We also try to match ethnic backgrounds. For example, if the couple were of Jewish background, then we would try to use a Jewish donor. If the couple were Oriental, we would pick an Oriental donor, and if the couple were black, we would use a black donor.

How is artificial insemination performed?

First we must pinpoint the day of ovulation, and this we are now able to do quite easily with certain chemical tests. Then we inseminate the patient on that particular day of her menstrual cycle and sometimes again on the next day. The sperm, which has previously been collected from the donor, is deposited within the cervix and may also be placed in a plastic cup that is kept over the cervix for several hours. Either live or specially frozen sperm may be used. Usually one to six inseminations are necessary. If the patient is not ovulating or has menstrual irregularity, these problems must, of course, be corrected before the insemination can be successful.

Couples who desire artificial insemination should not be hung up with religious or legal factors. The doctor is injecting sperm just as he would inject insulin or penicillin to treat a medical problem.

What about the recent successes in producing "test-tube" babies? Will this technique really help women with fertility problems?

This technique was developed for those women who have blocked fallopian tubes but whose ovaries and uterus are normal. The principles of the technique are simple. An egg is removed from the woman's ovary with a small instrument—the laparoscope—after hormones have been used to stimulate ovulation. This egg is placed in a special container and mixed with the husband's sperm in a special solution containing some of the mother's blood serum. Fertilization usually occurs with ease.

This fertilized egg is then maintained in appropriate tissue culture for approximately two and a half days. The major problem now is getting the product of the conception implanted within the uterus. When the fertilized egg is ½ to 1 millimeter in size, it is artificially introduced into the uterus, since the tubes leading from the ovary to the uterus are closed in these cases. While implantations have apparently been successful, we do not know if the doctors involved have completely solved the difficult step of implantation or whether these first children born in this fashion were only experimental accidents. These men are outstanding scientists, however, and they will soon report their techniques if they think they have been successfully developed. Then it will become relatively easy for more children to be born in this fashion.

Hopefully, sufficient funds will be made available for this type of research in this country.

7

LABOR AND DELIVERY

Why does the United States rank so poorly with regard to infant mortality? Some charts show that twelve or fourteen other countries have better infant survival.

These statistics are difficult to interpret because different countries use different criteria to determine what constitutes an infant mortality. Some countries don't keep accurate or complete statistics, and some don't count premature babies who do not survive.

Part of the explanation also involves the nonwhite population of the United States, which has a much higher incidence of heart disease, diabetes, high blood pressure, etc., which increase the risk of maternal and infant mortality. What's more, there are many areas in this country where poor blacks do not get proper prenatal care, although we are making progress in this regard.

If we used only the statistics on maternal and infant mortality among our white population, we would be right up there at the top of the world. I believe it is safer for a Swedish woman to have a baby in the United States than in Sweden, even though Sweden is at the top of the safety lists.

The three major causes of maternal mortality are infection, hemorrhage and hypertension, but deaths from obstetrical anesthesia are increasing in percentage as the three major causes decline.

What is the first sign of labor?

Abdominal pain is the most common sign that labor is about to begin. This pain is caused by the uterine contractions which will eventually expel the baby.

Two other signs of impending labor are a burst of amniotic fluid or a bloody discharge, which occurs when the protective plug which closes the cervix is being expelled. During the pregnancy, this bloody mucous material has prevented bacteria from the vagina from entering the womb and infecting the baby.

Any of these symptoms is reason to call the obstetrician so he can determine if it is time for the patient to enter the hospital.

What is false labor?

False labor is caused by painful and somewhat irregular contractions which do not lead to a gradual opening of the womb. False labor can usually be identified by the fact that there is generally no rhythm to the timing of these contractions, and they do not become progressively stronger.

If the contractions are occurring ten to thirty minutes apart, are relatively painless and are lasting only ten to fifteen seconds, the woman may be having what are known as Braxton Hicks contractions. These contractions, which can occur anytime during the last trimester of pregnancy, are efforts by the uterus to maintain good muscle tone and should be regarded merely as practice sessions for real labor. Braxton Hicks contractions account for almost all of the false alarms that doctors see.

It is not necessary to head for the hospital until the contractions have some rhythm and regularity and are occurring every five to seven minutes apart, even though what we first think are Braxton Hicks contractions may develop into true labor.

What causes a woman to go into premature labor?

This is a major obstetrical complication which we really don't understand, mainly because we don't understand labor itself. But we do know that certain problems seem to be involved—urinary-tract infection, hypertension, and a small amount of placental separation, which all tend to stimulate the uterus to begin its contractions. Premature labor also tends to occur more frequently in lower socioeconomic groups, for reasons we don't understand. Whether this has to do with chronic poor nutrition, inadequate development of the uterus and its blood supply, or anxiety is not known.

What can be done to halt premature labor?

Premature labor can be difficult to stop, although we do have several drugs that are often effective. While some physicians are still using intravenous alcohol to halt premature labor, this technique is not the most effective and is much more distressing to the mother since the effective dose of alcohol is very intoxicating. Although there are other very effective drugs now being used safely in Western Europe and South America, the F.D.A. is not yet allowing these medications to be used in this country except on an experimental basis.

If premature labor cannot be stopped, what are the baby's chances of survival? In other words, how small a baby can survive?

The baby's survival depends upon its weight and the conditions surrounding its birth. Premature babies who are delivered under optimal obstetric conditions have a 65 percent chance of survival when they weigh two to two and a half pounds, a 75 percent chance when they weigh three pounds, and a 94 percent chance when they weigh between three and four pounds.

The major causes of death among premature babies are injury during delivery, inadequately developed lungs, and infection.

If a woman wants to have her baby on a particular day, is it safe to have labor induced?

This elective induction of labor is one of the most potentially dangerous obstetric practices in the United States.

I realize that elective induction of labor is convenient for the obstetrician because the babies are born during the daytime. I realize it's convenient for the patient and her family to be able to make their plans on a definite schedule. But a woman may pay a considerable price and may take considerable risks when she has elective induction of labor.

First, there is the risk that the pregnancy is not as close to term as the physician believes. The baby's lungs may not be mature, and it may develop hyaline membrane disease, in which the lungs are unable to expand properly—a potentially fatal condition or at least an extremely expensive one, since the baby may require prolonged hospitalization.

Second, if the labor does not proceed well and the contractions are not rhythmical and progressively stronger, the obstetrician may have to administer larger and larger amounts of the medication, which is given intravenously to stimulate the labor. This medication can interfere with blood supply to the uterus, and the baby may develop oxygen starvation, which necessitates a difficult forceps delivery or even a cesarean section, both of which would probably not have been necessary if spontaneous labor had been allowed to develop.

Women must understand that labor is a complicated biological event. It's almost as if a combination lock has to be opened, with all the parts falling in place. We're not sure what all those parts are, but we do know that the gradual aging of the placenta causes increased irritability of the uterus, which sets in motion the mechanism that controls uterine contractions. The aging placenta also signals the adrenal glands in the fetus to produce the substances that cause the fetal lungs to mature. Then the placenta signals the fetus to produce the substance that stimulates labor. It's a complicated process, and many things must happen right on cue.

If a doctor induces labor, he is making an educated guess about when all these things are ready to occur. And he must give the mother a labor-inducing drug which has the potential to harm the baby. So if the induction of labor results in a difficult delivery or a cesarean section, the physician has probably made a mistake. If it results in a baby that is not in excellent condition, again the physician has probably been in error. In elective induction of labor, no obstetric problems should arise. The fetus should be ready to be born, with lungs fully matured. The fetus should be in the proper position, and labor should proceed normally and rapidly with no complications.

Women should be aware that the elective induction of labor is associated with some of the greatest maternal and fetal complications in obstetrics, although it can be performed safely if the obstetrician is extremely careful about the decision to induce labor and is with the patient throughout its course. Women should be very wary if their doctor sends his patients to a hospital where nurses start the Pitocin, the labor-inducing drug, and the physician remains in his office until labor is advanced and delivery imminent. This is to me unacceptable obstetric practice.

Are there times when it is proper to have labor induced?

Yes, there are, and these are called *indicated* induction of labor. Induction of labor may be indicated when the mother has high blood pressure or kidney disease, when the baby is in distress, or, very rarely, when the baby is overdue and the danger from its remaining inside the uterus becomes great. In this last case the obstetrician must ask himself, Is the baby safer in the nursery or in the uterus? The answer to this question is not always easy.

How can a woman protect her rights when she enters a hospital, so that decisions about her care are not forced upon her?

As we have already discussed, this matter should be settled with the obstetrician early in the pregnancy. Long before a woman is ready to deliver her baby there should be discussions concerning her wishes and preferences, and she should insist on retaining the responsibility for many of the decisions affecting her care after she enters the hospital.

I believe, for instance, that a woman has the right to decide whether or not she wants to have an enema. If she feels strongly against an enema, I think that is her prerogative, unless the rectum is quite full of feces. In this case, it is particularly important to have an enema, not only because the woman will be more comfortable but because the feces can prevent the baby's head from descending as rapidly as it normally would, especially if there is constipation.

I also think the woman has the right not to have her perineum shaved if she doesn't have an excessive amount of hair. (The perineum is the area between the vagina and the rectum.)

And I repeat, she has the absolute right to have her husband or partner present during labor and delivery unless there is some extenuating circumstance. Now I realize there are some husbands who are emotionally unable to participate in labor and delivery. Some men can't even watch the movies the obstetrician uses to educate couples concerning childbirth. Conversely, there are wives who would prefer that their husband not be with them during this time. Sometimes the wife doesn't want the husband or partner to see her in this "compromised" position, or she may feel the experience would be too traumatic for him.

Every woman should also have the right to select the type of anesthesia and analgesia which will be used during labor and delivery—provided she has no medical complications and her selection will have no untoward effects upon the fetus or the labor.

Every woman has the right to request that her baby be born without forceps if there are no problems or undue delay in the delivery of the infant. On the other hand, a woman must understand that the obstetrician has special expertise in these matters, and she should abide by his decision if he feels during the course of delivery that using forceps would be advantageous for the mother and the baby. The usual forceps delivery is gentle, actually protective to the child, and preferable to having the infant's head beat against a tough vaginal outlet.

It is entirely reasonable for a woman to request that no episiotomy be performed if it can be reasonably avoided. The episiotomy is an incision which is made to prevent tearing of the area between the vulva and the anus. But here, again, the woman should trust her physician's judgment and realize that he cannot, or should not, let her rip her perineum.

A correctly performed surgical incision heals well; a tear does not. Following an episiotomy the patient will have less discomfort and will not have damage to the sphincter muscle around her rectum, which could prevent her from having good control of her bowel.

A woman also has the right, and the privilege, to have her baby right after it has been born and resuscitated, to hold it close to her skin and to nurse it if she desires. She and her husband both have the right to share this very beautiful moment, fondling their newborn child together. It is also a nice idea, if the hospital routine permits, for the husband or partner to remain with his wife during the first night following delivery.

Let's step back a moment. What exactly happens when a woman arrives at the hospital?

Admission procedures vary in different hospitals, but they are generally designed for the comfort and convenience of the patient in labor. So she goes directly to the labor and delivery area while her husband, friend, or family goes to the admitting office without her.

Under ideal circumstances, the patient is placed in a private room. This room should have a pleasant decor and its own bathroom and shower so that the woman has the opportunity to take a shower if she wishes. She is given a hospital gown to wear, but if she is very, very early in labor, she can wear one of her own gowns if she chooses. This is generally impractical, however, because labor is associated with a vaginal discharge of considerable amounts of bloody mucous material.

Next the patient's history is taken by the nurse to determine if any complications or emergencies are present. The nurse will ask if the patient has been bleeding. Does she have a severe headache? Are her contractions occurring almost one after the other? Has she had a urinary-tract infection or has she had any burning or frequency of urination? Has she had a fever or chill? How long have her membranes been ruptured? Once the nurse has ascertained that there are no emergencies, the patient then has her blood pressure taken and is examined.

Who will perform this examination, and what will it include?

A nurse or a resident will perform a vaginal examination, similar to the examinations the woman's own doctor has been performing throughout her pregnancy.

This examination is important because it tells whether the mouth of the womb is open, whether the baby's head is high in the pelvis, or whether it has begun to descend into the birth canal. It also tells whether the baby is in a normal position and reveals whether the membranes (or fluid sac surrounding the baby) are ruptured or intact. Once the vaginal examination is complete, the resident or nurse will listen with a stethoscope for the fetal heartbeat. The rate will be carefully recorded. Then an enema may or may not be given.

Now the woman will be free to relax and await the progress of her labor. Whether she chooses to lie in bed or sit in a chair depends on her. If she prefers to lie in bed, she should lie on either side so that the heavy uterus does not cause pressure on the great vessels that supply the uterus, thereby reducing the oxygen supply to the fetus.

At what point should the obstetrician arrive?
The physician is contacted by phone after the patient has been examined. He is informed of her condition and the status of the infant. During the very early stages of labor, it is not necessary for him to be in the hospital unless complications exist or there is the likelihood of problems arising.

We generally expect the physician to come to the hospital when the patient is in good productive labor and the womb has dilated to about four or five centimeters, which is about one and a half to two inches. He should take complete charge and remain in the hospital through the completion of delivery. But even then, it is not necessary that he always be in the labor room. Indeed it is not even advisable. The patient and her husband or partner should enjoy a bit of privacy, with the physician available in the labor suite should they need him.

How can a woman make certain her physician will remain with her most of the time?
A candid conversation among the woman, her husband or partner, and the obstetrician early in the pregnancy is the only way to settle this question. The couple should learn the philosophies and policies of the physician. They should also ask how he conducts labor and what his feelings are about the different methods of pain relief.

Exactly what happens during the course of labor?
There are four stages of labor, although the first three are the most important. The first stage of labor involves the softening of the mouth of the womb, followed by its gradual and complete dilation to a size of about ten centimeters, or approximately four inches. By the end of the first stage of labor, the cervix, or mouth of the womb, has become as wide as the main body of the uterus. This usually requires six to ten hours, depending upon whether the woman has had previous children.

The second stage of labor begins when the cervix is fully dilated and ends with the birth of the baby. In women who have had previous children, this stage usually lasts about thirty to forty minutes. In women who have not had a child, this stage lasts an hour or an hour and a half. This is the most critical period of labor for the fetus, and it is essential that the fetal heart be appropriately monitored.

How is the fetal heart monitored?

There are three types of fetal monitoring. Two types consist of external and internal monitoring with the use of electronic devices. The third type of fetal monitoring is simply listening to the fetal heart with a stethoscope.

In external monitoring, a small, very sensitive microphone is placed on the woman's abdomen, right over the fetal heart, so that the physician can actually hear the heartbeat and record it. This fetal heart rate and its relationship to the uterine contractions lets us know whether the baby is in trouble, and this external form of monitoring is generally satisfactory in routine deliveries. However, when complications arise and the physician is concerned about the progress of labor or the condition of the fetus, he will want to monitor the fetal heart rate more accurately. Then it becomes important to use internal fetal monitoring, in which an electrode is attached through the vagina to the baby's scalp. This can be done without any injury to the baby or the woman, and it enables the obstetrician to measure very precisely the baby's responses to each uterine contraction.

Electronic fetal monitoring is one of the greatest advances made in obstetrics in recent years. In my own department at the University of Alabama, we are developing a very small computer that is attached to the fetal monitoring machine. This computer will predict during labor, with nearly 100 percent accuracy, those infants who are at risk and must, therefore, have careful and continuous internal monitoring.

Important as fetal monitoring is, however, we must not cause the patient to feel dehumanized by the use of an electronic device. She must always be treated with dignity and tenderness during this time.

What if the hospital does not have fetal monitoring equipment?

Then the obstetrician or the individual who is responsible for the labor should actually listen to the fetal heart with a stethoscope placed over the mother's abdomen. The physician should listen to the fetal heart every thirty minutes during the first stage of labor and after each contraction when the mouth of the womb is fully open. This technique is not nearly as accurate, however, because the human ear is not able to count rapid heartbeats or to perceive precisely the critical changes in heart rate that are related to uterine contractions.

What can be done if the labor is taking too long?

Let's first define what we mean by too long. A first stage of labor lasting more than twelve hours and a second stage in excess of two hours may be considered prolonged. Labor that is prolonged may be dangerous to the child since during each contraction the oxygen supply to the fetus is reduced.

We generally treat such prolonged labor with Pitocin, a medication which increases the strength of uterine contractions and reduces the interval between them. Pitocin should be used only when it is medically indicated and not merely for convenience. It should be used in conjunction with electronic fetal monitoring to ensure that the stimulated uterine contractions do not reduce the oxygen supply to the fetus.

If Pitocin is not effective it may become necessary to deliver the patient by cesarean section, since the fetus can tolerate for only a limited time the slight reduction in its oxygen supply caused by the uterine contractions.

What happens during the third stage of labor?

This is the period, lasting from five to twenty-five minutes, from the birth of the baby to the delivery of the placenta. It is a period of great danger to the mother because it is the time when potentially fatal hemorrhages can occur.

The major cause of obstetric hemorrhage is failure of the muscles of the uterus to contract and clamp down on the uterine blood vessels. If this happens, the blood pours out, and the patient can lose a quart of blood in a matter of minutes.

Other causes of obstetric hemorrhage include a ruptured uterus, a large baby, or a baby in an abnormal position which results in a tearing of the cervix or vagina. Obstetric hemorrhage is most common among older women, women who have had five or more children, and women who deliver twins.

Although we have medications to deal with these problems, obstetric hemorrhage remains a great threat. And if a woman has a severe hemorrhage following delivery, she stands a five times greater chance of infection because the loss of blood seems to change her immune mechanism. That is why we prescribe antibiotics to prevent serious infection in those women who have had a severe hemorrhage during delivery.

What happens during the fourth stage of labor?

This is the period, approximately one hour in length, after the placenta is delivered. During this time in a normal delivery, the uterus is still contracting so that excessive bleeding does not occur.

Many pregnant women have difficulty deciding whether or not to have anesthesia. How is this decision best made?

Every obstetrician should discuss obstetric pain relief with his patient during the course of the pregnancy, and he should explain what type of anesthesia is available. But I believe the woman herself should make the decision—provided, of course, she is not endangering her own health or that of her baby. I also believe the woman should make the decision about whether she will be awake or asleep at the time of delivery.

There are many women who feel they want no pain relief at all—even though there are no data to indicate that no medication is safer for the fetus than the small amounts that merely cause maternal relaxation. But there are women who are purists about this, and I respect their wishes. If they want nothing, it would seem quite reasonable that they have nothing.

Then there are women who have told me, "Although I really want to be awake, and I am extremely interested in participating in labor and delivery, when it becomes uncomfortable, give me a little something." These patients can receive small amounts of medication which will allow them to feel as if they have had several martinis. They are aware of everything that is going on, but they are more comfortable. As a matter of fact, many times a woman can participate in the labor more effectively this way. She is relaxed and not so frightened. She can carry out the proper breathing techniques, and she can push down more effectively without fear. In the absence of obstetric complications, such medication causes absolutely *no risk* to the fetus.

But isn't anesthesia dangerous to the baby?

This is one of the most controversial subjects in obstetrics. There are a number of pediatricians and obstetricians who say that any type of pain relief during labor will reduce the sucking reflex of the baby, make it sleepy, and interfere with the bonding process which occurs as mother and child cuddle and respond to each other after delivery. This is very difficult to determine, because bonding is such a complex phenomenon. A mother who is tense, ambivalent about a child, jealous of the child's effect upon her own freedom, concerned about what the child may do to the parents' relationship, may have no analgesia whatsoever and still have tremendous problems establishing a good mother-infant relationship. Her child will be nervous, have colic, and generally respond to her anxiety.

On the other hand, just because a woman is asleep at the time of the birth does not mean she is not going to become a fine mother. The infant may be a bit sleepy from the anesthesia, but in a very short time it will be totally awake, and mother and child can develop a beautiful, warm, loving relationship. Human infancy is such a prolonged period, unlike animal infancy, that it is quite possible that what happens during the first twenty-four hours of a child's life is not as important as some would have us believe.

Of course I would prefer that my patients have minimal amounts of analgesia so they are not completely narcotized and the fetus is not drugged. But in some women this is inhumane. They can't tolerate the discomfort of labor. So I believe the middle-of-the-road policy is the best. If the mother has the opportunity for preparation for childbirth, she should have the opportunity to decide what type of anesthesia or analgesia she should have.

I have delivered women who were completely asleep and whose babies were a bit narcotized because of the mother's inability to handle the labor. And I have seen these children grow up into beautiful, warm, loving adults. So I know from personal experience that it can be this way.

I remember very clearly one young woman whose own mother had died during childbirth. This patient, understandably, was fearful of labor, but she really wanted to have a child and eventually became pregnant. When she entered progressive labor, I gave her a small amount of analgesia and put her into a very tranquil sleep. I can remember very well which labor room this woman was in at the North Carolina Memorial Hospital and how comfortable she was and how easy her delivery was for her, although she was not awake. And I remember the excitement of her nursing the baby the next morning. This woman raised this boy to become an extremely good student, a great football player, and a delightful young man.

What are the safest types of anesthesia for childbirth?

There is no question that the safest method of pain relief for delivery is a pudendal block with nitrous oxide. Here the obstetrician blocks the nerves going to the vulva, just as a dentist would block the nerves going to the lower portion of the jaw. If a woman intermittently receives no more than 50 percent nitrous oxide and 50 percent oxygen (the air we breathe contains only 20 percent oxygen) she will have an extremely pleasant feeling. The birth can occur either naturally or by outlet forceps, and the baby will not be narcotized at all because nitrous oxide merely replaces the nitrogen in the baby, and will not cause it to be asleep. Moreover the child eliminates the nitrous oxide during the first five minutes after birth.

The next safest method of anesthesia is probably the spinal block. Although the spinal is used throughout the country for all types of operations, it is subject to special problems when used in delivery. If not given in careful amounts, it may cause a fall in the mother's blood pressure resulting in a reduction in oxygen to the fetus.

The spinal must be administered by a competent obstetrician or anesthesiologist just as the baby is about to be delivered. The mother must be given a sufficient amount of fluids intravenously so that her blood volume is expanded, and she should be given only the smallest dose of anesthesia that will be effective. Her blood pressure must be monitored every thirty seconds during the first five minutes, and if it begins to fall, a medication (ephedrine) must be given to counteract the problem.

Spinal anesthesia should never be given merely to slow down the course of a labor until the obstetrician is able to arrive at the hospital. Unfortunately, this does happen. But a good obstetrician is with the patient after she enters productive labor, so there is no need to slow down labor awaiting his arrival.

Another type of anesthesia is epidural anesthesia. It differs from spinal anesthesia in that the anesthesia is not placed in the spinal canal, but rather in the spinal column in the space surrounding the nerves. It can be used to relieve the pain of labor, whereas spinal block should only be used at the time of delivery. The epidural block causes the nerves which leave the spinal column to become anesthetized.

These particular nerves contain the sympathetic ganglia, which are the small nerves that control blood pressure. So again, epidural anesthesia must be administered carefully to prevent a fall in blood pressure or a reduction in the blood supply to the fetus. But when used properly, the epidural can be the Cadillac of anesthesia. The patient is free of pain, awake, not completely paralyzed, and able to participate in the birth of her baby.

What is a paracervical block?

This form of anesthesia is injected around the cervix. Since the pain of uterine contractions travels from the uterus through the cervix and then into the nerves which lead to the spinal column, if we block the nerves around the cervix we can cause tremendous reduction in pain from uterine contractions.

But there are certain dangers here, too. If excessive amounts of the anesthetic are used and absorbed into the mother's circulation, there can be reduction in the blood flow to the fetus, a very dangerous thing, as we have already discussed. The paracervical block must be given carefully. There must be at least a ten-minute wait between injections and only very dilute solutions must be used. This block should not be used in premature labors or when there may be a reduction in the fetal oxygen supply.

Is it safe for a woman to be totally asleep under general anesthesia at the time of delivery?

Because there are certain major dangers, I am opposed to having women asleep under general anesthesia unless it is absolutely essential for some medical or psychological reason. One of the greatest dangers in being asleep is the possibility of inhaling vomitus. When a woman is in labor, she ceases her digestive processes so that food and secretions remain in her stomach even though she has not eaten for ten or twelve hours. When she is put to sleep, there is always the possibility she may vomit. If she inhales this vomitus into her trachea, she and the fetus stand a good chance of dying—the baby from lack of oxygen and the mother from a chemical pneumonia caused by the very acidic contents of her vomitus.

I am generally opposed to the use of general anesthesia for vaginal delivery unless there is good reason. For instance, sometimes there is fetal distress when the infant does not receive enough oxygen, and the delivery must be accomplished quickly. Then putting the mother to sleep is the safest thing to do. There are other times when major hemorrhaging demands quick delivery of the baby, and again putting the mother to sleep is the preferable method. But whenever general anesthesia must be used, the mother should be "intubated." That means that she should have a tube placed down her trachea so she can remain well oxygenated and not inhale any of her gastric contents.

Despite the dangers, some women still prefer to sleep through the whole labor and delivery.

It is true that some women are so frightened they want to be completely knocked out. While this is not desirable, it certainly is the patient's privilege, provided she understands the risks involved. There are also some physicians who find this technique preferable.

I think you can divide these physicians into two groups: one is really concerned about the patient's discomfort, and is willing to have the patient in a tranquil sleep for this reason; the other group wants its patients pretty well knocked out so the doctor doesn't have to spend prolonged periods in the hospital. Sometimes obstetrics is practiced this way, and women who are pregnant must be aware of this.

What else can you tell us about fetal distress?

As we have discussed, this term is used when we are afraid the baby's well-being is in jeopardy, usually from a reduction in its oxygen supply. Normally the baby's heart beats between 130 and 160 times each minute, and this heartbeat remains pretty constant, even when the uterus contracts. Although the contraction does cause a reduction in the uterine circulation, there is sufficient oxygen reserve within the fetus so that the heart rate doesn't change. During the second stage of labor, however, just prior to delivery, the baby's head pushes against the bottom of the vagina, and this head pressure may cause a reflex to occur throughout the baby's vagus nerve, which is one of the large nerves of its body. This reflex may result in a slowing of the baby's heart rate, and with electronic fetal monitoring equipment, the physician can make this diagnosis very easily. He can watch the baby's heart rate improve soon after the contraction disappears on the monitor, so he knows that this problem is not dangerous. It is caused by the temporary pressure on the head and not by a diminishing oxygen supply.

A more ominous problem, however, is called a late deceleration. Here the slowing of the baby's heart begins after the contraction is already in progress. This means that the baby is not tolerating the contraction as well as it should because of an insufficient reserve of oxygen.

We treat this problem by turning the mother on her side and giving her oxygen. We also get ready for a possible cesarean section, in case the decelerations continue and the baby continues to have difficulty.

There is a third, or variable, type of deceleration, and this occurs when the baby's umbilical cord is being compressed during the contraction. We can diagnose this problem quite clearly on the electronic monitor because the heart rate begins to fluctuate almost as soon as the contractions start. Here, too, a cesarean may be necessary, depending on the severity of the problem.

In both the late and the variable decelerations, we have a method for determining the condition of the fetus. Working through the vagina, we make a small nick in the baby's scalp and take a bit of its blood. This sample is then analyzed for its oxygen content as well as its acidity. This is not in any way dangerous to the fetus or the mother. Although it can be a bit awkward and takes some skill on the part of the doctor, this test prevents us from performing many unnecessary cesarean sections. Often we find that although there are variations in the heart rate, the baby's oxygen supply is good, and it is really not in any distress or jeopardy.

Another possible indication of fetal distress is the presence of meconium in the mother's vagina. This meconium is the thick, green first bowel movement of the baby. It is always passed when the baby is being born buttocks first, but it may indicate fetal distress during headfirst birth. For this reason, the passing of meconium always requires that the fetus be monitored internally.

Should anesthesia be given during premature deliveries?

In premature births, I would prefer that the mother receive no type of analgesia or anesthesia whatsoever. I've had the experience of having to alter agreements with women who wanted to be asleep during delivery but who went into premature labor. When this happened, I had to sit down with these women and say, "Now we have to work together to have this baby, and we just can't afford to give you or the child any type of pain-killer other than a local block for the delivery. We don't know why the premature labor is starting, and we don't want to create additional problems." When you sit down and talk to women like that, you get marvelous cooperation because they know you are on their side and working as a team. Of course, the husband is included in the discussion so that he understands the situation too.

When is it necessary for a baby to be delivered by forceps?

Forceps have gotten a very bad name because they were previously used for very difficult deliveries. Today these deliveries have been replaced by the cesarean section, and forceps are now used mostly to help ease the baby's head through the outer portion of the vagina. This can be a very helpful and very safe procedure if the baby is not born spontaneously, as most are. The use of such "outlet forceps" can shorten the second stage of labor and therefore much of the discomfort of labor by fifteen to thirty minutes.

I should also mention that there is another type of forceps which is used when the baby's head is still an inch or more inside the vagina. These *midforceps*, as they are called, are used to pull the baby through the vagina, and sometimes it is necessary for the obstetrician to rotate the baby's head into proper position. If not performed with great skill, this procedure can pose some risk to the infant's brain.

Do forceps cause birthmarks?

Not as a rule. The forceps may cause some imprint on the baby's face, but this will last only a short time.

What are some of the major reasons that women require a cesarean?

One in ten deliveries today is performed with the operation known as cesarean section. In this operation a surgical incision is made through the abdominal wall into the uterus. It usually takes only five or ten minutes until the baby is removed, but it may require a full hour to close the abdomen.

The major reasons women require cesarean sections are problems with "the three *p*'s"—the passenger, the passage, and the power of uterine contractions. The baby, or passenger, may be too large or may be in an abnormal position, such as feet or face first. The passage, or the bony pelvis, may be too small or improperly shaped to allow safe passage of the baby. Or the uterus may be incapable of producing adequate power in its contractions to push the baby through the birth canal.

A cesarean section may also be necessary because of such conditions as fetal distress, obstetric hemorrhage, or medical complications such as diabetes, hypertension, and so forth. The thoughtful obstetrician will explain these problems to his patients and indicate just why a cesarean section is necessary.

A woman who requires one cesarean section will probably be advised to have sections for her other pregnancies. The uterus is weakened by the incision, and the scar could rupture under the stress of future births. There are considerable data, however, to indicate that vaginal delivery is safer for the mother and baby than a cesarean if the reason for the previous section is no longer present. However, the threat of malpractice, the increased fee for a section and the fact that the repeat cesarean section can be done at a convenient time for the obstetrician and patient have not allowed the dictum "once a section always a section" to be broken.

Haven't cesareans increased in recent years?

Yes, for several reasons. First, we have come to realize that a cesarean is preferable to a difficult forceps delivery, which can be hard on both mother and baby.

Second, thanks to fetal heart monitoring, we are better able to diagnose fetal distress, so we are aware of babies who are getting into difficulty, and we perform cesarean sections, which prevent these babies from being born vaginally with cerebral palsy or other afflictions.

Third, we have found that one of our most difficult obstetrical problems involves breech deliveries, where the babies are born feet or buttocks first instead of headfirst. Breech deliveries are best performed by cesarean section. Breech babies have the highest incidence of cerebral palsy, particularly among premature babies, because the umbilical cord sometimes collapses during labor and the fetus suffers lack of oxygen. Another problem with the premature breech baby is that it tends to get its head caught in the cervix during delivery. The body gets through all right, but the head, which is larger than the trunk in the premature breech, is trapped. The baby may suffer a fracture of the neck or damage to the liver or the spinal column. So more and more obstetricians have come to believe that most premature breech births are best delivered by cesarean section. The full-term frank breech (where the buttocks come first) may generally be delivered through the vagina unless there are other complicating factors.

Finally, the elective induction of labor often results in cesarean sections, the majority of which could have been avoided if spontaneous labor had been allowed to develop. The threat of malpractice suits has also increased the number of cesarean sections.

An emergency cesarean can be particularly upsetting if a woman was planning to have natural childbirth.

It is understandable that such a woman might be deeply disappointed and frustrated. She might feel that she has somehow failed in her role as a mother, and if the father is unable to be present at the cesarean delivery, she might feel that she has let him down too. At the University of Alabama we try to soften this disappointment by at least allowing the father to watch the child being born by cesarean section.

If the cesarean is an emergency procedure and the woman is shocked and saddened by this change in plans, she should talk freely and openly about her feelings as soon after the operation as possible. With the proper support from her physician and partner, including an explanation of the potential dangers had the cesarean not been performed, she will find that even a cesarean birth can be a joyous occasion.

What is the best type of anesthesia for a cesarean?

I believe general anesthesia is usually preferable. Although spinal and epidural anesthesia may be given, the spinal may cause a fall in blood pressure with all the accompanying dangers we have discussed. Falls in blood pressure are less likely with epidural anesthesia. This is an excellent anesthesia if skillfully given.

Under ordinary circumstances, and in all cases of fetal distress, it is preferable for a skilled anesthesiologist or nurse anesthetist to use general anesthesia—first by giving a small dose of sodium pentothal, which is a barbiturate, and then giving the mother a paralyzing agent plus nitrous oxide and oxygen. This paralyzing agent is used for two reasons: so that a tube can be placed down the patient's trachea so that she can breathe safely and will not choke on any vomitus, and so that her abdomen will become more relaxed for the operation.

Doesn't sodium pentothal put the baby to sleep?

No, it doesn't, and for a very interesting reason. The pentothal which is injected into the mother's bloodstream circulates throughout her entire body, and only the small amount of pentothal which is in the blood supplying the uterus gets across the placenta to the fetus. What's more, part of this medication is absorbed by the uterus and the placenta, so most of the mother's tissues protect the baby. If only 250 to 300 mg of pentothal are used and the obstetrician delivers the baby within five to ten minutes, the mother will be asleep and the baby awake.

The same principle applies when the mother receives pain-relieving drugs during labor. The mother's body absorbs the great majority of the medications; thus the fetus receives very little sedation.

What causes stillbirth?

Many, many factors are involved in stillbirth. The problem may be associated with maternal infection that may affect the baby or the placenta. Or, stillbirth may be caused by maternal heart disease, high blood pressure, kidney disease, diabetes, or hemorrhage from the placenta.

On very rare occasions, a difficult forceps delivery and difficult breech extractions can cause injury so the baby dies during delivery.

I can't think of anything more tragic than losing a baby, either at birth or soon after delivery.

Neither can I, and it is normal and necessary for parents to feel intense grief following the loss of a newborn infant. Nevertheless it is sad, but true, that our society offers less emotional support during this tragic period in a couple's life than after any other type of death in their family.

The best advice I can give to such bereaved parents is to mourn openly as they would for any other relative. They should, if they desire, touch or even hold the dead infant so that the death becomes a reality to them. They should verbalize their anguish to each other and to close family members and friends. And if they would like to talk with another couple who has experienced a similar loss, they should request that their physician make the necessary arrangements.

It may take weeks or even months for the couple to reach the point where their grief is bearable, and that is why I believe that they should wait at least six months before attempting to have another child.

Home deliveries seem to be coming back into vogue. Do you ever sanction these?

I feel that home deliveries are putting obstetrics back fifty years. I do, however, feel that the hospital environment must be made more like the home, where the spouse and family members can be with the patient and provide support at this very important time.

Let me tell you a few case histories which explain why I feel the way I do about home deliveries. A number of years ago, after I finished my tour in the army, I had a six-month period before I could go back into the residency program at Johns Hopkins. So I decided to do some general practice in Zebulon, North Carolina. That was in 1947, and most of the deliveries around Zebulon at that time took place at home.

I'll never forget one particular case in which a husband came for me in his car after his wife had been in labor four or five hours. I rushed home with him and found his wife about three fourths through the labor. Since we were going to deliver the baby in bed and we wanted her to help with the process, we gave her very little analgesia. The delivery occurred spontaneously with no problem at all—not, that is, until the patient began bleeding profusely. Her placenta had only partially detached from the uterus, and blood began to pour out of her vagina as if it came from a water faucet.

If we had been in a hospital, we could have had a catheter placed in her vein to replace some of the fluid she was losing. Blood would have been sent down to the blood bank for cross-matching, and additional physicians would have been present to assist me.

No such help or facilities were available, so I put my hand up into the uterus and attempted to remove the placenta manually. It was very adherent and very difficult to remove, and it was perfectly obvious to me that I was leaving small pieces inside the uterus. The patient continued to bleed, so I placed my fist against the mouth of the womb in an attempt to slow the bleeding by exerting pressure. Then I used all the medications I had available in an attempt to make the uterus contract. But the patient still bled alarmingly.

The nearest hospital was about twenty-six miles away, but I felt it was important to get there. We put the patient in the back seat of their car, and all the way to the hospital in Raleigh, North Carolina, I massaged this woman's uterus and compressed the vessels of her womb with my hand in her vagina. The bleeding continued, and I was afraid the woman was going to bleed to death before we arrived at the hospital.

Fortunately, we did arrive in time. We got fluid and blood going and were able to scrape out the parts of the placenta that remained. The patient survived, but what had started out as a simple home delivery had turned into a nightmare. Had we not been able to get this woman to the hospital when we did, she would have died.

Another frightening case occurred in the middle of the night on one of the muddy roads around Zebulon. This time the patient was a woman who was doing reasonably well during the initial stages of labor, but then the contractions seemed to get slower and slower, and farther and farther apart. If I had been in a hospital, I would have had medication and equipment which would have allowed me to treat her safely. At home, however, my management of her labor was severely compromised. Labor remained poor, and I considered taking the patient to the nearest hospital, eighteen miles away over very poor roads. As the contractions became slower and slower, the fetal heartbeat dropped almost to nothing. If I was going to save this baby, I was going to have to do a difficult forceps delivery in bed without anesthesia.

And that's what I did. It was certainly one of the most difficult things I've ever done in obstetrics. It was difficult for the patient to cooperate. I did not have anesthesia or sufficient light. And when the baby was born—barely breathing and with a very slow heartbeat— I did not have the proper instruments to carry out the resuscitation. Somehow I managed, and the baby survived. But again it was a touch-and-go situation in which I was extremely fortunate. Had I been in the hospital, these problems would have been easily overcome.

So the fact is we can never predict when there are going to be catastrophic things happening in obstetrics. During labor we can be enveloped by a huge tidal wave of complications that can wash everything right out to sea. You may think there won't be any complications, but they swoop down on you all at once. These two patients had no problems whatsoever during pregnancy or early labor. Then suddenly we had two near-catastrophes—one involving the mother and the other involving the child.

I remember an extremely tragic situation where a home delivery resulted in a child's having cerebral palsy. This delivery was performed by another physician in Zebulon. Here a problem developed in which the placenta separated, and the baby did not have sufficient oxygen. It took the doctor one hour to get the patient into the hospital to complete the delivery. By that time the baby had suffered tremendous deprivation of oxygen, and today that baby is a severely handicapped adult. Had this complication occurred in a hospital, the baby would have been extracted in a matter of minutes by a cesarean section and would not have been damaged. Fortunately, Zebulon has an excellent hospital today.

How do you feel about the trend back to midwives?

That depends on the qualifications of the midwife. A nurse midwife who has received very special training is perfectly competent to perform normal deliveries, and can be a superb assistant to an obstetrician when major complications are present. But a nurse midwife is not to be confused with the lay midwife who has never attended a nursing school, has not received adequate obstetric training, and is not able to recognize the major obstetric problems or deal with emergencies should they arise.

How is the nurse midwife trained?

The nurse midwife has graduated from nursing school and passed the state boards and often holds a master's degree. This person has had at least two years of general nursing experience plus another nine to twelve months of training in a nurse midwifery school. This is intensive training in which the nurse midwife is taught prenatal care, nutrition, and the physiology of labor. Under careful supervision, the nurse midwife has the opportunity to attend a number of women in labor, to deliver their babies, to provide postdelivery care; and is taught how to perform pelvic examinations, breast examinations, and screenings for cancer. So the nurse midwife is an educated and highly skilled person who becomes an important member of the obstetric team.

Ideally, such a person should work with a group of obstetricians and should be responsible for the majority of prenatal care. If the nurse midwife is a woman, she can answer another woman's questions far better than a man, and she can be responsible for teaching preparation for childbirth.

I support the movement and have three nurse midwives working in my department. These are extremely competent women, and they have added a very personal dimension to the service. It is hoped that by their example, they will show the residents and medical students techniques to make women more comfortable and how to communicate better with patients in labor. These midwives provide normal prenatal care and supervise normal labor and delivery. But they always have an obstetrician as a backup in case a problem arises.

I believe the nurse midwife is going to have an expanding role to play in obstetrics in years to come. I believe the midwife will work more and more with groups of obstetricians and with high-risk patients, and, I predict, will work increasingly in rural hospitals, where there may not be trained obstetricians available and where nurse midwives will be totally responsible for labor and delivery.

Is a family doctor an adequate obstetrician?

Yes, provided he has had adequate training. Many physicians have had only three months of medical-school obstetrics training, and that's insufficient. On the other hand, there are family physicians who took six or eight months of obstetrical training and they have practiced for many years and have become extremely skillful. It's not so much a matter of whether the doctor is a family physician or an obstetrician, but whether he is vitally interested in delivering healthy babies and has had adequate training. Unfortunately you can't anoint a doctor and make him an obstetrician. It takes specialized training and experience.

Of course, as we have already noted, women who have special problems, such as diabetes, heart trouble, etc., should seek the services of a high-risk specialist.

What are your reactions to the technique called "birth without violence"?

This is a method of delivery also known as the Leboyer technique, which attempts to make the birth process as pleasant as possible for the new baby and enables the baby to adjust very gradually to its new surroundings outside the womb. The child is delivered in somewhat subdued lighting, so it is not exposed to the very bright lights of the delivery room. The infant is placed in a basin of warm water which is the same temperature as the amniotic fluid that has been its environment for the past forty weeks. With this technique, the baby doesn't feel such an extreme change. (Incidentally, our delivery rooms are way too cold; they are kept that way for the comfort of the obstetric team, but they ought to be about eighty degrees for the comfort of the baby.) Then the child is taken out of the water, wrapped in blankets, and laid to its mother's breast.

This is a nice way of letting the baby be born, but we must not develop a cult about this—just as we must not develop a cult about preparation for childbirth and a cult that says a woman must not have any pain-killer during childbirth. Each delivery is an individual matter, and there should be no hard and fast rules. It's a matter of using common sense.

One more thing about the Leboyer method. There are not the slightest data to indicate that this method of childbirth is going to make any difference in the child's IQ or future development. Leboyer is a nicety, not a necessity in obstetrics. But it should be available if parents want it. I personally feel that the infant would be just as happy if it was put next to its mother's skin instead of in the warm water.

I should also mention one *disadvantage* about the Leboyer method: if the lights are too low, the physician may be unable to see as well as he should. If a complication arises, he may not be immediately aware of it.

There is much discussion these days about postpartum depression. Are there physical reasons for this common problem?

Every obstetrician has observed postnatal blues many times. In order to understand what is happening, we must realize that during pregnancy a woman's body has become adjusted to high levels of estrogen and progesterone. Then, with delivery, there is a sudden fall in these hormones to a level that is actually lower than normal. Since the brain responds to hormone levels, this causes a woman to feel overly tired and to want to sleep and rest during the first few days after delivery. So it is normal for a woman to feel slightly irritable because of the fatigue of labor and the sudden tremendous reduction in hormones.

On the other hand, if a woman finds herself extremely depressed, this is not normal. This means she is having difficulty accepting her baby and its effects on her life, her independence, and her relationships within the family.

Some women, who didn't grow up in a family where there were

small babies, feel very insecure with newborn infants. When these women realize that they are going to have to bathe, dress, and care for this tiny person, they can become depressed.

Other women become depressed because the pregnancy was unplanned and unwanted. They would really have liked to have the pregnancy aborted, but social or religious pressure would not allow it.

Then there are women who are not happy in their marriages. They are insecure in their relationship with their husband or partner, and now another small human being may interfere even more with that relationship.

Why do some new mothers have psychotic breaks?

These women have generally had previous emotional problems. Although they may have been able to function without treatment, the added emotional stress of new motherhood is too much for them to bear. Some attempt suicide or even attempt to kill the child.

One of the most distressing things for a physician is to have a patient who cries hysterically, "I'm afraid I am going to kill my baby. I'm afraid I am going to kill my baby!" Indeed, the child must be taken from such a mother because this is a serious emotional problem, and therapy is necessary.

Another psychotic break involves schizophrenia, where the patient withdraws totally from reality. She doesn't know where she is, she doesn't realize she has had a child, she doesn't know her husband, and she lies in a trance. The problems of assuming responsibility for the child are so great that she breaks with reality because that is the only way she can handle the stress.

Good prenatal care should have ferreted out those women who have psychological problems. Appropriate discussions should be held with the physician or some counselor so that the necessary adjustments can be made prior to the birth of the baby.

When can intercourse be resumed after the birth of the baby?

A woman should not resume intercourse for at least two weeks after delivery. If there has been an episiotomy, intercourse should not be resumed for two and a half to five weeks. Thereafter, intercourse may be resumed if it is not uncomfortable.

How soon after delivery does contraception once again become necessary?

Ovulation usually occurs between the fourth and sixth week following delivery. If the woman is going to use oral contraceptives, they should be started two weeks following delivery so she will be protected. We do not, however, recommend oral contraceptives for the nursing mother, because the pill may interfere with the milk supply. It is preferable for the couple to use condoms and jelly until nursing has ceased—or until an intrauterine device can be inserted, which can be done about six weeks after delivery. The diaphragm can be fitted three weeks after delivery without difficulty.

Breast-feeding goes in and out of fashion. What are the pros and cons?

The debate over whether or not to nurse one's baby becomes highly emotional. There are those who believe that every woman should try to nurse her baby, and if she doesn't, she is not a good mother and the emotional development of her child may be jeopardized.

Of course, it is preferable for a woman to nurse her baby. It is pleasurable for most women and for the child. A nursing mother can be sure the baby is getting adequate amounts of fluid, proteins, vitamins, and antibodies. But again we don't want to develop a cult about this. We don't want to insist that all women nurse their babies or make those women who don't wish to nurse feel guilty. If a woman wants to, that's great. If she doesn't want to, she doesn't have to. Infant formulas have been developed that are essentially the same as breast milk, and research may soon provide formulas with more immune factors to protect the baby than exist in the mother's own milk. So women should be encouraged, but not forced, to breast-feed.

And if problems arise and the woman is unable to nurse, she should have an honorable exit and not feel that she is a failure.

What advice can you give the woman who is worried that she won't be successful at nursing?

A woman who chooses to nurse her baby should be given special instruction and great support from her obstetrician and his staff. There are tricks to nursing and one of them is to be relaxed. So if a new mother has proper instructions, she is going to feel more secure about what she is doing, and this will be half the battle.

The new mother should also be given a list of names of other mothers who have nursed successfully, whom she can call during the weeks or months she is nursing so that she can ask any questions which arise.

Is it true that a woman who is breast-feeding is unable to become pregnant, that she is protected by a natural kind of birth control?

Women who are breast-feeding their babies do have suppression of ovulation and fertility. This is nature's way of protecting the baby's food supply, because if the woman were to become pregnant, her breasts would dry up and her infant could not survive. That is why breast-feeding provides very effective contraception in primitive societies, where it is not uncommon for women to nurse their babies six or seven times a day for two or three years.

Breast-feeding is not very effective in Western societies, however, because of the manner in which it is done. It generally takes about six sucklings a day to suppress ovulation. So when a woman begins to breast-feed her baby fewer than six times each day, when she starts giving the baby a bottle and solid foods, she should presume that she will be ovulating very shortly. She is signaling her pituitary gland and ovaries that her baby is growing older, and since it's nature's job to produce as many children as possible, fertility returns.

If American women nurse their children as do primitive mothers, by giving the baby little water or supplementary food until natural weaning occurs, pregnancy will occur very infrequently during the period when they are nursing.

8

ABORTION

Where do the current laws stand today with regard to abortion?

In January 1973, the Supreme Court repealed all abortion laws in this country. Up to the thirteenth week of gestation, a pregnancy may now be legally terminated in any state of the Union by mutual consent of the patient and her physician. A pregnancy may also be terminated up to the end of the second trimester (or twenty-sixth week) of pregnancy in accordance with guidelines established by the individual states. These guidelines have been established to safeguard the health of the mother. Nevertheless, there are still some physicians who refuse to perform abortions under any circumstances and there are still some hospitals which will not allow them.

How many abortions are performed in the United States each year?

It is believed that approximately 900,000 legal abortions are now performed in the United States annually. It is impossible to estimate accurately the number of illegal abortions performed annually prior to 1973, but the figure may possibly have been as high as 400,000 to 500,000.

The word "abortion" engenders such strong feelings. How did you, as a physician, come to grips with the dilemmas involved?

It was a slow and thoughtful process that took me many years. I was born and raised in Zebulon, North Carolina, a small town where my father was an elder in the Methodist church, and my mother was a deeply religious woman who impressed upon me as a young boy that illegitimate pregnancies and abortions were not things that nice people talked about.

I was thirteen years old when I first saw the birth of a baby. I had accompanied my father, who was a country doctor, on a house call. Just as we arrived, the patient delivered a premature infant in bed. I remember how impressed I was with the beginning of a new human life. On that day, no one could have convinced me that I would ever terminate a pregnancy.

Later, during my medical-school years at the University of North Carolina and at Johns Hopkins, abortion was seldom mentioned; it was used as a last resort to prevent a woman from dying during pregnancy. And I saw no more than four or five abortions during the five years of my residency training.

It is interesting now to remember how I felt when one of my classmates got a student nurse pregnant and then had her pregnancy terminated by a criminal abortionist. I could sympathize with him and understand his anxiety, but I remember seeing him in the hall several times and thinking, "I wonder how he did it; I wonder how he brought himself to take her to an abortionist."

It was not until many years later that I began to understand.

What made you change your mind?

The longer I was in practice, the more I encountered the serious problems, and sometimes even horrors, of unwanted pregnancy. I remember how shocked and saddened I was at the University of North Carolina when I conducted a careful survey and found that the majority of the pregnancies among patients in the lower socioeconomic groups were unplanned and unwanted. I was also disturbed by the disproportionately high number of infant mortalities and birth defects among these unwanted, unplanned babies. But I was not yet ready to become pro-abortion.

I began an enthusiastic program of disseminating family-planning information and developed a number of contraceptive-study projects. My efforts, however, were relatively unsuccessful.

For this reason, I next became an enthusiastic advocate of tubal ligations and vaginal hysterectomies for sterilization. Indeed, I was probably too enthusiastic for many of my peers, but I joined a lay group attempting to lobby and persuade the legislature of North Carolina to liberalize its laws concerning sterilization.

It was not until 1964, however, when I was asked to attend an international symposium sponsored by the Royal College of Obstetricians and Gynecologists in Australia, that I made my decision. Following the symposium, I traveled to Thailand, India, and Egypt as a lecturer in family planning and oral contraception. It has been a number of years since this trip, but the memories will forever influence my thoughts and professional activities.

What I saw were millions and millions of people at the poverty level who were overwhelmingly burdened with excessive parenthood. The hospitals in Thailand were inundated with women being treated for the complications of criminal abortions, and it became apparent to me for the first time that our methods of family planning must be backed by some safe system of abortion.

In India, the population problem was even more apparent. As I traveled from the Dum Dum Airport to the center of Calcutta, the roads, streets, and alleys were crowded with humanity. The next morning I took a three-block walk around my hotel. On this short walk, I saw three people lying in the street. They had died during the night, and their bodies were small and shriveled. No one knew they were dead; possibly no one cared. Down the street I saw two stretcher bearers making their solitary rounds to pick up the dead before the rats, crows, and flies could further foul the air.

There were masses of people, but there were no laughs and no smiles. The Hindu superstitions concerning the sanctity of life were apparent. Life, life, life was everywhere, but little happiness, little hope, only great sorrow and great famine.

The problems in Egypt were not much less. I saw one of the most tragic sights of my entire life in a small Egyptian village where the children sat quietly whimpering. Flies buzzed around their faces and landed in the corners of their eyes to eat the pus that was encrusted on their infected eyelids. The children were too exhausted to push the flies away.

Finally I came to the conclusion that man does not have the luxury to live in a world of unrestricted fertility. My trip had made it abundantly clear: abortion is a necessity. It is a poor second choice to contraception, but it is better than no choice at all.

I came to the realization that reverence for life must include concern for the quality of life of the children who are born as well as consideration for the rights of women unwillingly pregnant.

Because of their religious and moral convictions, many people believe that abortion is murder.

I realize that some people do have such convictions, but I firmly believe that one should not impose one's religious or moralistic beliefs on others by law, although it is perfectly proper to attempt to change another person's views by simple persuasion. Furthermore, Christianity, as it has been practiced for many centuries, does not always consider the killing of a human being as an act that is intrinsically wrong or immoral. The majority of Christians believe that some wars are necessary and that the taking of a life to protect one's home or loved ones is justifiable. So we can't really rule out abortion on religious terms.

What's more, it is my firm belief that women in lower socioeconomic groups suffer most from restrictive laws concerning abortion, and that is certainly an immoral situation. Rich women with know-how and financial means obtain safe, legal abortions, while poor women bear unwanted children or are butchered by back-street abortionists. So in my opinion, abortions are necessary under certain conditions for the emotional and physical health of the women involved.

Moreover, legal abortion decreases the number of unwanted children, battered children, child abuse cases and possibly subsequent delinquency, drug addiction and a host of social ills believed to be associated with neglectful parenting. Legal abortion also decreases the tragedy of children born with serious birth defects.

Tragic as these cases may be, that is not adequate justification for the destruction of human life.

There remains considerable controversy over the question of when life actually begins and when "ensoulment" occurs. Aristotle felt that the soul was infused on the fortieth day after conception in males and on the eightieth day in females. St. Augustine and St. Thomas Aquinas also decided that ensoulment did not occur at conception but at a later date. The controversy of ensoulment was settled for Catholics, however, by Pope Innocent XI, who established by papal ruling that the soul was infused at the moment of conception. This is the view held by the "right-to-life" movement.

One can make a strong argument that a person is not a person until he or she has developed a personality. The mere fact that a human fetus can move, respond to stimuli, breathe, and sneeze makes it no different from the chick, turtle, baboon, or rabbit fetus, all of which can do the same.

Some people feel that abortion is only one step removed from euthanasia.

Although determining the end of human life is as difficult as determining its start, abortion and enthanasia are separate issues. And one step does not necesarily lead to another. We set speed limits at 55 mph., and that does not necessarily mean we are going to move them to 65. Legal abortions have been performed in Japan and Central Europe for over twenty years and they are no closer to euthanasia than we are.

But who speaks for the fetus and its right to live?

The question over whether the fetus is a person is unresolvable. But nowhere in the United States can a fetus claim legal rights of property, inheritance, or damages until it is born alive. Those who argue that the fetus has the right to life from the moment of conception are giving the fetus a right which no born person shares—the right to use another person's vital organs. No one has the "right" to use my kidney, to receive some of my blood, etc., unless I specifically allow it.

Surely society has a responsibility to uphold its moral integrity.

I believe it is the moral responsibility of society to protect a woman's right to control her own body and to determine the timing and extent of her own fertility. Men and churches have for too long controlled women's femininity, sexuality, and reproductivity.

But doesn't legalized abortion encourage promiscuity?

Fear of pregnancy is notoriously inefficient as a deterrent to sexual behavior, as we discussed in regard to the pill.

Is a husband's permission required for an abortion?

No. The spouse's consent is often requested, but not required. I remember one case where this consent became a problem. The couple was seething with hostility when I entered the examining room. The wife said, "Doctor, I want an abortion, and my husband won't let me have it."

He replied, "I don't believe in abortion."

The wife countered, "I am forty-five years old, and I don't want another child. We already have four. I love them very much, but I refuse to have another child. Besides, at my age I am running a great risk of having a mongoloid child."

The husband got up, looked out the window and said, "I don't give a goddamn."

I entered the conversation. "Let's see if we can't reconcile these points. First, if you are forty-five years old, there is no question that you do run a very high risk of having a child with Down's syndrome, or mongoloidism. In the general population, this problem occurs only about 1 in 1000 pregnancies, but in your age bracket, it occurs almost 1 in 50. However, we now have a test we can perform which will tell us whether you are carrying a child with Down's syndrome. In this test, known as amniocentesis, we would obtain some of the fluid which surrounds the baby and then grow these cells and study their chromosomes. Although there are never any guarantees, this test is extraordinarily accurate. And we can perform it for you."

The wife still insisted, "I refuse to have this baby."

The husband still replied, "I refuse to sign for an abortion."

I suggested that this couple go home and discuss this matter in their own home. I did explain to the husband, however, that we would perform the abortion without his permission if necessary because recent court rulings had granted the wife the right to make this decision. I felt, however, that the couple should make this important decision together for the sake of the marriage, and I hoped that he would agree to a termination of the pregnancy if this was what his wife really wanted.

The woman looked at her husband with great determination. "Henry, we have four lovely children; but we're having a terrible time making ends meet now. I don't know how we're going to educate the children we have already. You know how you fret and become angry when I have to skimp on the grocery money at the end of the month. Why do you want another child?"

They finally agreed to go home and talk things over, and by the time they returned the next day the husband had changed his mind. The decision was made in favor of the quality of life of the present family rather than the "right to life" of the embryo. This type of decision is always difficult, but it should be made by the couple themselves and not by others in society who impose their own moral convictions.

This case illustrates the real dilemma of the abortion issue: Can women choose to abort babies they don't want and the country doesn't need or must every effort be made to raise to maturity every conception? The abortion argument continues with great fury because there seems to be no "middle ground."

Is parental consent necessary for an abortion to be performed on a minor?

The necessity for parental consent varies from state to state. The age of legal consent in Alabama is fourteen; in other states, it is eighteen to twenty-one. Most physicians would prefer to have parental consent if a teenager is involved, whether or not such consent is required by law. But we recognize that there are circumstances where this would be impractical or not in the best interest of the patient.

What are your own criteria for performing an abortion?

Basically I am willing to perform an abortion for any woman who has carefully weighed all her options and who has come to the conclusion that a termination of her pregnancy is in her own best interest.

I must repeat that I feel that abortion is a poor second choice to contraception or even sterilization, but it is better than no choice at all. The decision to terminate a pregnancy is neither casual nor easy. Still it is a necessary decision for many women. There are far too many unwanted children and unhappy mothers in this world. And I can tell you dozens of stories about women who have died or nearly died as a result of dangerous, criminal abortions. For this reason I have worked to eliminate the legal, social, and cultural restraints that have prevented women from having safe, therapeutic abortions and sterilizations when they want them.

If a woman is considering an abortion, where can she turn?

If she has a gynecologist, she should discuss this matter with him as soon as she suspects she is pregnant. If she has no personal physician, she can turn to her local Planned Parenthood organization, to a local medical school, or to a major community hospital. It is not necessary to be referred by a doctor.

What type of psychological counseling should a woman have before deciding on an abortion?

A physician, social worker, or gynecological nurse specialist should encourage the woman to express her feelings freely about this pregnancy. What are her reasons for not wishing to have this child? Are these reasons temporary or correctable? Is the woman expressing her own honest desires regarding abortion, or is she merely acquiescing to the desires of her husband or other relatives?

Every woman seeking an abortion should be advised of the options which exist in her circumstances. She should be told that during the pregnancy she can find safe and helpful refuge in one of the Florence Crittendon or Salvation Army homes if she needs such help. She should also be advised that she can put the child up for adoption if she feels she is totally unable to keep it.

There are many faces of women who seek therapeutic abortions. Some come in terror. Others come with the look of hope or expectation that an enormous burden will be lifted from them. And then there are women who softly cry or sob. These are the women who really tug at your heartstrings so that you hear yourself ask over and over, "Are you absolutely sure this is what you want? It's not too late to change your mind."

There are other times when I am struck by the callous, matter-of-fact attitude of some patients. These women look upon a therapeutic abortion with the same emotion that they feel for a tooth extraction. A short time ago I was interviewing a very well dressed lady about thirty-five years old who simply said, "Doctor, I am So-and-so's mistress. I am pregnant, so let's get it over with." The name she dropped without hesitation belongs to a well-known national figure who indeed would need to have his mistress abort any pregnancy. There was no remorse, regret, or complaining. This woman refused any sedation so she could catch the evening flight back to Washington.

Teenage abortions seem doubly disturbing because the pregnant female is herself almost a child.

The story is, indeed, often sad among the fourteen- to nineteen-year-old age group seeking abortion. These young girls are beset by two of the greatest disappointments that any woman can have: the realization that the man they love, who fathered their child, does not give a damn about them, and the recognition that their hopes and expectations of marriage and motherhood have been thwarted. Well over 50 percent of all the teenagers I have aborted have had their hearts broken by boy friends who cruelly ask, "How do I know the baby is mine?" or "You stupid fool, why didn't you do something to keep from getting pregnant?" Other young men bluntly state, "I'm too young to get married. I have too many things that I want to do."

I remember so well one teenager who came for her abortion accompanied by both parents and by her young lover. This young girl was crying and almost in shock. She looked at me like an animal who had been caged or cornered. The parents were very anxious for me to proceed with the termination, but I needed more time to decide if this was what the patient wanted. I went over to Debbie, put my arm around her, and said, "Debbie, you are my patient. I am delighted that your parents are here showing support, and I appreciate your boy friend being brave enough to come with you. But I want you to tell me that you want an abortion, that this is your decision and that it is not based on what your mother and father want but what you yourself really desire."

Her response was simple. "Doctor, I'm too young to get married. I know that now. I didn't mean to become pregnant. I didn't know that I could. I felt Johnny and I were in love, but I want to finish my education and I just don't feel I can have a baby."

Debbie was a child being aborted. She had succumbed to television and movie glorification of sex. She had no knowledge of contraception, and she found herself living a horrible nightmare. As we prepared to terminate the pregnancy, Debbie pulled out a small teddy bear from a large purse and snuggled it as she was sedated.

What are the different methods of abortion?

The methods of abortion depend mostly upon the stage of the pregnancy. The simplest and earliest form of abortion involves menstrual extraction, in which the menstrual fluid and contents are sucked out of the uterus through a small tube. This type of abortion can be performed within two weeks after the first missed period.

Another technique which can be performed up to the twelfth week of pregnancy involves a simple suction curettage in which the physician injects some local anesthetic around the cervix, dilates the mouth of the womb and cleans out the contents by the use of a strong vacuum. This procedure can usually be performed on an outpatient basis.

Still another type of abortion, which can be performed during the thirteenth to eighteenth week of pregnancy, is known as a dilation and evacuation, or D&E. In this technique the mouth of the womb is dilated, the fetus is removed with ovum forceps and the remaining contents of the womb are removed by suction or scraping. This is the most difficult and dangerous abortion technique unless it is performed by a gynecologist with extensive experience.

Abortions performed between the eighteenth and twentieth weeks of pregnancy are also complicated, and there are five or ten times the number of complications than occur in earlier terminations. Hospitalization is required, and many patients actually go into labor and experience the emotional trauma of delivering a fetus that weighs ten or fifteen ounces. These later terminations also cause the greatest psychological stress for the physician and nurses because the fetus has identifiable structures.

Exactly how are these later abortions performed?

There are several different types of midtrimester terminations.

One method frequently used between the eighteenth and twentieth weeks is the injection of a very concentrated salt solution into the amniotic fluid surrounding the baby. The injection of this saline solution causes almost immediate death of the fetus by producing severe injury to the placenta and its vessels. The saline also initiates uterine contractions, which are minor at first but gradually increase in tempo after twelve to twenty-four hours. Labor generally begins between twenty-four and forty-eight hours following the injection.

The safest type of midtrimester abortion involves the injection of urea and a bodily substance known as prostaglandin, an extremely interesting compound which is essential to life. Prostaglandins were first discovered in the 1930s, but they have only recently become available for scientific investigation. They are present in almost all tissues of the body and are essential for urination, smooth-muscle contraction, peristaltic movements of the intestines, and the initiation of labor. If prostaglandins are introduced into the fluid surrounding the fetus or injected into the muscles of the womb, they gradually cause the muscles to contract and initiate labor.

Often a pencil-shaped piece of root of a Japanese seaweed is introduced into the mouth of the womb approximately twelve hours prior to the use of the urea and prostaglandin. This laminaria, as the seaweed is called, absorbs water from the surrounding tissues and expands in size about three to five times. This expansion causes the mouth of the womb to dilate and stimulates the uterus to begin contractions. After the laminaria has been in place for approximately twelve hours, a needle is introduced through the abdominal wall into the fluid surrounding the fetus. The urea and prostaglandin are injected into this fluid, further stimulating the uterus to contract. Another substance, known as Pitocin, is then used to augment the contractions. The pregnancy is usually terminated in eight to sixteen hours.

How late in a pregnancy can an abortion be performed?

At the University of Alabama, we do not perform abortions after the twentieth or twenty-first week of pregnancy unless there is a life-threatening condition affecting the mother or a fetal abnormality which has been documented by amniocentesis. We take this position because it is difficult to determine the precise stage of a pregnancy, and the fetus may be more developed than we realize. It may, in fact, be born alive.

What are the major complications of abortion?

Complications depend on the type of abortion. The suction curettage, performed only during the first twelve weeks of pregnancy, has relatively minor complications of infection and bleeding.

The major complications in later terminations involve hemorrhage, premature rupture of membranes, and postabortal infection.

Abortion, like childbirth, is associated with potential risk. But if the physician is competent, fewer than 1 percent of the patients will have complications of bleeding, infection, or perforation of the uterus. This is the same risk that exists if the mother goes to term and delivers a child in the hospital.

When is it necessary for a woman to have an abortion for medical reasons?

It is common for an abortion to be performed if an amniocentesis reveals a defective fetus or if a pregnancy results from a rape that was not properly treated with the morning-after pill. But it is extremely rare that some life-threatening medical condition of the mother requires an abortion.

The recent advances in obstetrics and the care of the newborn allow most women to carry a pregnancy to the point where the child stands a good chance of surviving. If a baby can be delivered weighing three pounds and is undamaged in the delivery process, there is a 90 percent chance that the child will survive and be healthy.

Obstetric patients who have major medical problems, such as diabetes, impending heart or kidney failure, severe liver disease, or even malignancies, may be hospitalized or kept at home on total bed rest. With proper medical and nursing care, the majority of these women can carry their pregnancies to the point where the fetus could survive outside the womb. However, this may happen at great sacrifice to the mother. In addition, it may become necessary for the baby to be delivered prematurely, and the patient may be faced with a hospital bill of up to $10,000, or could you believe $50,000?

Will having an abortion affect the woman's ability to have future children?

The opponents of abortion have published a great deal of data to indicate that abortion causes prematurity and other obstetric complications in future pregnancies. Good data are not available in this country, and part of the misunderstanding stems from the fact that most of the information we have on abortion was collected before the Supreme Court decision, during a time when safe abortions were difficult to obtain and when physicians were still in the process of learning proper techniques and safeguards.

Nevertheless, the effect of abortion on prematurity or miscarriage in future pregnancies is an important subject. Those of us who have been associated with large numbers of abortions in a medical school have not yet seen any indication that a relationship exists.

What are the mortality rates in abortion?

The mortality rate of therapeutic abortion in the state of New York is approximately 5.6 per 100,000 procedures. The mortality rate is 2.9 when the pregnancy termination is done prior to the twelfth week and 21.1 per 100,000 if it is done after that period.

These later statistics are almost identical with the maternal mortality rates in the United States, which are approximately 20 per 100,000 deliveries. So we can say that the risk of mortality from a midtrimester abortion by saline injection or prostaglandin is approximately the same as the risk involved in completing the pregnancy and giving birth.

Have you encountered many psychological complications following abortions?

It has been my experience that psychological reactions to the procedure are usually minimal—provided, of course, the woman had no serious emotional problems to begin with.

This subject is discussed in depth by Drs. Howard J. Osofsky and Joy D. Osofsky in *The Abortion Experience* (New York: Harper & Row, 1973). The Osofskys found that the psychological problems associated with the legal termination of pregnancy were much less than the psychological and emotional problems of patients who requested abortions but were denied. If I may quote: "Patients who were denied an abortion because of insufficient psychiatric problems fared considerably worse post-delivery than did the apparently more emotionally disturbed individuals following abortion.

"Age, marital status, education and number of children have important effects on patients' attitudes. Catholics have experienced somewhat more difficulty with decision-making and guilt than have non-Catholics. Individuals undergoing a second-trimester abortion have more difficulty in decision-making and more post-abortal feelings of guilt and depression than individuals undergoing a first-trimester abortion. However, it should be emphasized that negative feelings have been uncommon among all groups, and that among individuals with follow-up evaluations, patient satisfaction has been high."

The Osofskys also found that "post-abortal blues" were usually short-term and mild if a woman had no serious emotional problem before the abortion.

We should also note that *denying* a woman a therapeutic abortion can inflict significant psychological consequences on her and the child. The best study in this regard involved a twenty-year follow-up on 120 children born to Swedish women whose request for abortion on psychiatric grounds had been denied. There was a control group of children who were of the same sex and born in the same hospital immediately after delivery of the unwanted children. The data indicated that the unwanted children had not had the advantage of a secure family life during childhood; they had registered more frequently for psychiatric services; they had engaged in more antisocial and criminal behavior; and they had received more public assistance.

How long does it take to recuperate from an abortion?

This will depend on the type of procedure performed. A patient can return to work the same day following a menstrual extraction, the next day following a suction curettage, and three days after a midtrimester abortion.

What should an abortion cost?

For a menstrual extraction, the most simple form of all abortions, the cost is about $100.

A termination of a pregnancy during the first 6 to 12 weeks generally costs between $150 and $175. A termination of a pregnancy after the 13th week up to the 20th or 21st week, may cost from $400 to $600. Abortions performed later than 21 weeks, although not usually recommended, can run as high as $1000.

9

STERILIZATION

How do you regard the growing trend toward sterilization?

I have always felt that women should have the right to control their own sexuality and reproductivity even though men and their religions have kept women from this right until recent years.

When I was a resident in the 1940s, the majority of hospitals required a woman to have at least eight pregnancies before she could be sterilized by tubal ligation. Each hospital had its own specific formula based on age and number of children before sterilization was allowed, but the decisions were made by physicians and committees, rather than by the women themselves.

Now that times have changed, I have only one hard and fast rule as a gynecologist: the decision for sterilization should be made by the woman, with or without her husband's consent. I believe there should be no firm restrictions based on a woman's age or number of children.

I believe that sterilization can be a reasonable solution to the side effects of the pill and IUD. Sterilization can also serve as an alternative to the inconvenience of the other forms of contraception. But sterilization may be a nonreversible decision which must be made thoughtfully. If there is any doubt at all, I always urge the woman to use some nonpermanent form of contraception because I feel it is extremely important for a physician to protect the patient against herself. On several occasions I have refused to perform a permanent sterilization because I felt the woman was either too young or not emotionally prepared to make such a decision, and later a number of these women have come back to thank me.

I remember one very attractive twenty-five-year-old woman who was separated from her husband with whom she had already had one child. The couple had had a terrible fight. The husband, who was a heavy drinker, had three mistresses in three different locales. When the wife found out, the couple separated. The wife became disgusted with men, and she was certain she would never want to marry again or have children.

Because she was young and attractive and might meet somebody else and later want to become pregnant, I prevailed upon this woman to use a nonpermanent form of birth control. Then, no more than three months later, my projection began to come true. She met another man, divorced her husband, married this new man, and had another child. I now see this woman once a year, and she always thanks me for not allowing her to have a sterilization when she was so upset.

I have had other young patients who have asked for sterilization because they were frightened of using the pill or IUD. Again I have been able to talk these women out of this procedure by suggesting other effective, temporary methods of contraception, such as the diaphragm; and subsequently a number of them have decided to bear children.

What factors do you consider most important in deciding to perform a sterilization?

I would be strongly influenced to perform a sterilization if a couple clearly dislikes children and clearly does not wish to make the adjustments entailed in raising a family. Other considerations might be the size of the family a couple already has and the state of the woman's health. If a pregnancy would jeopardize a woman's life, her health, or even her reasonable sense of well-being, that would be reason to perform a sterilization.

By and large, I am very reluctant to sterilize a woman soon after a divorce or broken love affair. I am also reluctant to sterilize a single woman, although here again there are no hard and fast rules, and I recently sterilized a young Ph.D. who was only twenty-six years old. She had never been married or pregnant, but her background thoroughly convinced me that she did not like or want children.

I am also reluctant to sterilize a woman whose husband has some serious health problem. If he were to die at an early age, she might some day wish to remarry and have another child—although at the present time, with her first husband still alive, she might insist this could never happen. In situations of this kind, I believe it is more appropriate to sterilize the partner with the shorter life expectancy, if that is possible.

A particularly difficult decision involves those couples who are still in their twenties, who have a stable marriage with only one or two children, but who believe they want no more. Here the physician must listen carefully to their views, point out the alternatives to sterilization and allow them to make their own decisions.

Another situation where sterilization brings tremendous emotional relief involves those young couples who have had children born with serious birth defects. Even though genetic counseling can sometimes offer some reassurances, many of these people are terrified of having another abnormal baby, and for their peace of mind, sterilization is sometimes the best approach. I had one twenty-three-year-old patient who was married at the age of eighteen and who had two abnormal children. Although her third child was perfectly normal, this young mother and her husband had developed an incredible fear of future problems. There was no way they could be reassured, and sterilization of this woman, despite her young age, had a greater effect of binding a marriage than any other sterilization I've ever performed.

Of course, sterilization is not to be recommended for every couple who have had one or even two abnormal babies. Genetic counseling should always be the first approach in these matters.

Where do you stand on sterilization of the retarded?

It is difficult for me to comprehend the philosophy that people with severe mental retardation should be allowed to have children. It has been my experience that people with severely limited intelligence simply do not make adequate parents, although there is certainly no reason they cannot enjoy their own sexuality.

Unfortunately our laws today make it very difficult and expensive for sterilization to be performed on the severely retarded. A community sterilization committee must be formed and court proceedings must be initiated since a court order for sterilization is required. This, of course, can be very expensive and often prohibitive, especially for members of the lower socioeconomic groups.

It is not necessary to go through all this red tape, however. A vaginal hysterectomy can be performed if it is proven that a retarded patient has menstrual dysfunction and is unable to take oral contraceptives successfully. So mothers of mentally retarded teenagers should understand that this procedure is available, even though many physicians are reluctant to operate on the mentally retarded because of the fear of a lawsuit.

The need for thoughtful and practical regulations concerning the sterilization of the mentally retarded is urgent. This is obvious from the following case history.

Mary Lou is a cerebral palsied, mentally retarded young woman of twenty who is bedridden. She receives welfare assistance and her mother works when possible. The mother pays a "baby sitter" to take care of Mary Lou when she is away, but this person is unreliable.

This mentally incompetent young woman has been impregnated three times by boys in the neighborhood who look for the opportunity to enter the house when Mary Lou is not protected. She has been aborted once and has given birth to two children.

The mother has gone to see poverty lawyers for help but she has found three obstacles: first, the lawyers do not want to take a sterilization case because it is controversial; second, Mary Lou is not twenty-one and therefore cannot be sterilized without a court order; third, the mother cannot get a court order without being able to pay the legal fees.

The sterilization of the mentally retarded is a delicate issue. If parents of retarded children are willing and able to protect their children from pregnancy and to provide for them and their offspring with life trusts, there is no problem. But rarely is this possible, and the parents of mentally retarded girls are desperate for help; they spend a great amount of their time and energy caring for these girls and protecting them from pregnancy.

What's more, the children of the retarded are rarely adoptable, since few people are willing to bear the cost and accept the responsibility of caring for these children. Each mentally retarded child on welfare costs the government, and therefore the people, $50,000 if the aid is extended to age seventeen; however, the figure is usually much higher because these offspring are often subemployable and must be assisted much of their lives. It is not unusual for the institutional care of a mentally retarded child to cost over $250,000 during his or her lifetime.

Does sterilization affect a woman's sex life?

For many women, enjoyment of sex actually increases after sterilization because the fear of pregnancy has been removed.

Tubal ligation does not involve the ovaries, uterus, or vagina, and the woman's hormones, sexual arousal, and orgasm are not affected. She will continue to menstruate, and she may develop the same menstrual problems as women who have not had tubal ligations.

How are sterilizations performed in women?

Sterilizations, known as tubal ligations, are performed in one of two ways: either through the abdominal wall or through the vagina. In either case, the object is to close the fallopian tubes, by either burning, tying, or clamping them shut, so that any egg which is released from the ovary cannot unite with a sperm to cause pregnancy.

The easiest time to perform an abdominal sterilization is following a delivery or a midtrimester abortion (thirteen to twenty weeks), when the enlarged uterus is very close to the surface of the abdominal wall. If a small abdominal incision is made, about two and a half to three inches long, the physician can insert a small instrument and rotate the uterus from side to side in order to reach the fallopian tubes.

He can then cut the tubes in one of several ways. The most foolproof method of sterilization is known as the Irving procedure. Here the physician ties the fallopian tubes in two places, cuts between the ties, and implants one end of the tube in the wall of the uterus, creating a blind end. Once this is done, there is no way a pregnancy can result, and we have found the Irving procedure to be 100 percent effective.

Another type of sterilization is known as the Pomeroy tubal ligation. Here the fallopian tubes are grasped by an instrument, tied with plain catgut, and then cut in two so that, once again, an egg can no longer pass through. This is an extremely simple procedure. It can usually be done in twenty-five minutes; the catgut dissolves in several days, leaving a space between the two ends of the tubes.

Still another type of sterilization is called a laparoscopic tubal ligation, and this is the "bellybutton," or "Band-Aid," procedure that has attracted so much attention. In this technique, the abdomen is filled with carbon dioxide, a harmless gas, so the physician has a better view of the abdominal contents. The laparoscope is inserted through a small incision in the navel. The surgeon locates the fallopian tubes and makes a second, small incision to insert another instrument with which he will burn (cauterize), cut, or place a clip on the fallopian tubes. This procedure is quite rapid, taking little more than thirty minutes. The majority of patients sterilized through the laparoscope can go home the same day.

A newer technique of sterilization with the laparoscope utilizes an ingenious plastic ring or clip which fits very tightly around the fallopian tubes, much like a rubber band. This tubal clip can be applied very quickly and is gaining in popularity in the United States because it seems to allow reversibility in 50 percent of patients.

Is abdominal sterilization painful?

If the woman is put to sleep, she will, of course, suffer no pain, although she may have some minor postoperative nausea and discomfort. Laparoscopy, or buttonhole surgery, involves less postoperative pain because less healing is involved, but the woman may suffer some shoulder pain because the gas that is used to distend the abdomen accumulates in the upper abdomen, producing a referred pain to the shoulder. If the gynecologist uses only local anesthesia for the abdominal surgery, there may be some discomfort during the operation, but here the complications of general anesthesia are avoided.

METHODS OF STERILIZATION

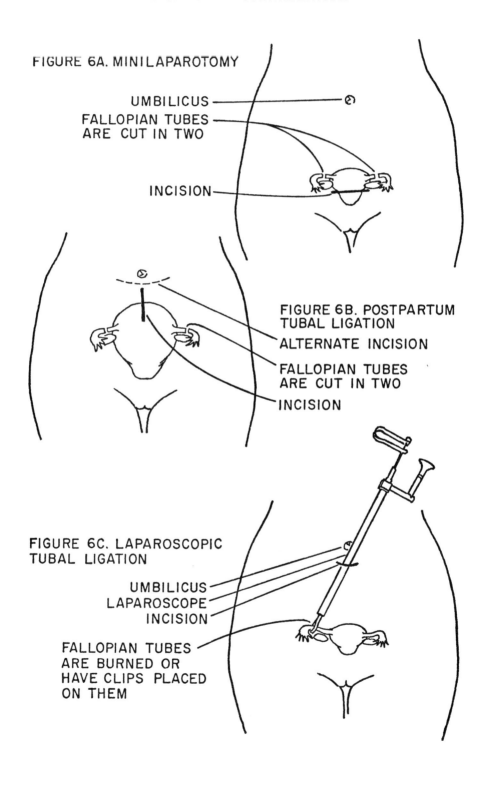

FIGURE 6A. MINILAPAROTOMY

UMBILICUS

FALLOPIAN TUBES
ARE CUT IN TWO

INCISION

FIGURE 6B. POSTPARTUM
TUBAL LIGATION

ALTERNATE INCISION

FALLOPIAN TUBES
ARE CUT IN TWO

INCISION

FIGURE 6C. LAPAROSCOPIC
TUBAL LIGATION

UMBILICUS
LAPAROSCOPE
INCISION

FALLOPIAN TUBES
ARE BURNED OR
HAVE CLIPS PLACED
ON THEM

How much hospitalization is required after a tubal ligation?

This depends on the type of surgery. Many women who have a laparoscopy are able to return home the same day, but the more traditional methods of tubal ligation require a hospital stay of several days. A newer form of abdominal sterilization is called a "minilap." A small incision three inches long is made transversely above the pubic bone.

Are there ever any complications with tubal ligation?

All operations involve some risk, and sterilization procedures, which require entry into the abdominal cavity, are no exception, although statistically the risks are small. The woman could have bleeding of the skin or inside the abdomen. Depending on the skill of her surgeon, she may suffer burns if her tubes are cauterized; this is now very rare because of the development of new instruments.

Following tubal ligations, patients may acquire an infection with symptoms of fever and severe pain, and in rare cases they may develop a drug reaction to the anesthesia. The greatest risks of any sterilization procedure involve the use of general anesthesia.

How are sterilizations performed vaginally?

In this procedure, the gynecologist cuts through the thin piece of skin in the back portion of the vagina in order to gain access to the fallopian tubes. Then he merely puts on a tubal clip and closes up the vagina; the whole procedure can be completed in less than ten to twenty minutes. The patient usually stays in the hospital for twenty-four hours because of postoperative pain.

There is a note of caution here, however, because this technique should only be performed on a woman whose uterus is freely movable. It should not be attempted on one who has pelvic inflammatory disease, endometriosis, or adhesions, as it will usually be unsuccessful.

What are the possibilities for complications in vaginal sterilization?

Statistics indicate a higher rate of infection and bleeding than in abdominal tubal ligation. But the duration of hospitalization and discomfort is less.

How effective is tubal ligation? What is the pregnancy rate?

Approximately 1 out of 600 women having these procedures becomes pregnant. The failure is usually due to the two ends of the tube reconnecting.

What about cost?

The costs vary according to the geographic locale, the type of operation, and the amount of time the woman spends in the hospital.

If the sterilization is performed on an outpatient basis without general anesthesia, the hospital will often charge a flat fee of about $150 to $200.

If the woman remains hospitalized overnight, the cost will be about $250, plus the use of the operating room (about $75), the anesthetist's fee (about $75), the use of the recovery room, and the cost of drugs. The physician's fee will range anywhere from $300 to $500. A laparoscopic tubal ligation will usually cost $750 to $1000, but it is covered by the majority of comprehensive insurance policies. If a woman is already in the hospital following an abortion or birth of a baby, her length of stay may be increased by about two days, and her physician will add a charge of $150 to $250 for this procedure.

Is it true that vaginal hysterectomies are sometimes performed as a means of sterilization?

Yes, it is, and this can be an acceptable technique for those women who are greatly bothered with moderate-sized fibroid tumors, precancerous lesions of the cervix, severe menstrual cramps, excessive bleeding, and premenstrual tension and fatigue.

If a woman desires sterilization and has bothersome menstrual problems, there is no point in her suffering four or five days each month with such menstrual difficulties—provided she can have a hysterectomy very safely.

While I do not feel one can justify doing an *abdominal* hysterectomy for sterilization, the vaginal hysterectomy can generally be performed in the same amount of time as the tubal ligation, thirty-five to fifty minutes.

In the last four years, thanks to antibiotics, we have had no major complications in over 350 vaginal hysterectomies performed for sterilization at the University of Alabama. One of the most satisfied patients I've ever had in this regard was a thirty-year-old divorced stewardess. All her life she had had an aversion to having children, but she had developed a very normal sexuality. She had severe menstrual cramps and pain and excessive menstrual flow. It would have been unreasonable merely to perform a tubal ligation when a vaginal hysterectomy not only freed her from her fear of having children but completely eliminated her gynecological problems.

It is absolutely essential, however, that the patient understand what is happening. Many women have a fixation about the uterus, and we men who are gynecologists must respect this. We must understand that having a uterus, even though it might not be used to have a baby, is culturally important to some women. When a woman is having an elective hysterectomy for sterilization, it is extremely important that all these matters be discussed. But on the positive side, some of my happiest and most pleased patients are woman who have had vaginal hysterectomies which accomplished sterilization and relief of their menstrual problems.

If a woman has only a tubal ligation, is it possible for her to change her mind and later have her tubes reconnected so she can once again become pregnant?

If a woman has any doubts or reservations about losing her ability to bear children, she should use some other, more temporary, method of birth control. Although fertility can be restored in 50 to 60 percent of those cases where the tubes have not been burned, sterilization is often irreversible.

I have had a number of women ask me for this sterilization reversal for very legitimate reasons. One thirty-two-year-old patient had had two children and wanted no more when she decided to have a sterilization. But one of her children died of leukemia and the other was severely handicapped in an automobile accident. Fortunately the operation to reconnect her tubes was successful, and she was able to have another child.

Another case involved a widow with five children who remarried. This woman's new husband had never had any children, and she earnestly wanted to bear his child. Here again we were able to reverse her sterilization. Before this microsurgery was performed, however, fertility studies were performed to make certain the woman was still ovulating and was able to conceive and bear children.

It should be understood, however, that the operation to reverse sterilization is not a simple one. It requires about four hours of operating time and is quite expensive.

When would you suggest sterilization of the male partner?

I believe the same criteria should exist for a man contemplating vasectomy as we have already discussed for a woman considering tubal ligation. Here again, the surgeon must protect the man against himself. There are some extremely macho men whose ability to father children is important in maintaining their ego. On the other hand, there are other men who feel, as many women do, that limiting the number of children is important.

Careful discussion is once more important, but I do not believe it is necessary for a person—man or woman—to obtain his or her partner's approval. Of course, I encourage patients to discuss this matter openly and thoughtfully, but each individual has the right to control his or her own body, and it is not up to the physician to obtain consent from the partner of the person being sterilized.

What actually happens in a vasectomy?

This is a very simple surgical procedure in which a small incision is made in the man's scrotum in order to reach the tubes, known as the vas deferens, which carry the sperm from the testicle up through the prostate into the urethra. A small piece of each tube is removed and the severed ends are sealed off. The incision in the scrotum is closed with no visible scar. Although the male will continue to produce sperm in his testes, these sperm, which comprise a very small part of the ejaculate, will be prevented from reaching his semen and from being expelled. The man will continue to have the same amount of ejaculation and there will be no less pleasure, although it will be impossible for him to cause a pregnancy.

A vasectomy takes about twenty minutes and can be performed in a doctor's office, a clinic, or a hospital. A local anesthetic is used.

The technique is much less complicated than sterilization of a woman; therefore the incidence of complications is much lower. The man might experience some temporary swelling, pain, or minor infection, but the discomfort is short-term.

How will a man's sex life be affected?

There should be no effect at all on a man's capacity for arousal, erection, orgasm, and intercourse, provided he has a good healthy attitude about sex. If he has had some previous problems of impotence, however, or uncertainties concerning his male identity or sexuality, a vasectomy may aggravate these psychological problems.

Urologists have been shot, they have received threatening phone calls, been kidnapped and molested by individuals who blame their sexual problems on either a vasectomy or a circumcision performed by the physician. That is one reason urologists are extremely careful about screening candidates for vasectomies.

Is a man completely sterile after the operation?

Not for a while. It takes about twenty ejaculations for the man's semen to become completely free of sperm, and another method of birth control must be used to prevent an unwanted pregnancy during this initial period. It is essential that the patient return to his physician as directed after the operation to determine whether his semen is sperm-free. No male should consider himself sterile until his physician informs him this is the case.

What is the failure rate in vasectomies?

About 1 in 600 cases—approximately the same as in female sterilizations.

What if a man later decides he wants to father a child? Is a vasectomy reversible?

Some success has been achieved in recent years in reconnecting the male tubes, but the chances are small. A man should not consider sterilization unless he feels certain he wants no more children.

What should a vasectomy cost?

From $150 to $300.

10
VAGINITIS AND BLADDER DISORDERS

VAGINITIS

Could we talk now about the problems of vaginal discharge and vaginal itch? What causes them?

These symptoms, which are often lumped together under the term *vaginitis*, have many causes: infection, hormonal deficiencies, improper cleansing habits, allergies to soaps and deodorants, or even emotional upsets, which can change the chemical balance of the vagina.

We know that vaginitis is more common among women who are overweight or pregnant and in women who are taking antibiotics and oral contraceptives. We also know that some vaginitis is caused by a normal, but heavy, vaginal secretion, which can be irritating and create problems of its own. Careful diagnosis is essential so that treatment can be tailored to the specific problem involved.

Women should realize, however, that not all vaginal discharge is abnormal. The glands in the vagina, cervix, and uterus all produce their own secretions, so if a discharge is clear in color and not irritating or foul-smelling, it is probably within normal range. The time for concern is when there is a sudden change in the type or amount of discharge or if there are accompanying symptoms of irritation or odor.

Why do some women go along for many months with no problem and then suddenly develop severe vaginitis? Does this mean they have picked up a new infection?

Not necessarily. There are many types of bacteria growing in harmless amounts in the "normal" vagina, and these bacteria are constantly changing in type, number, and virulence. They may change because of fluctuations in hormone levels and the menstrual cycle. They may change in response to diet. And they may change because of other bacteria that have been introduced through the vagina.

Probably most important of all, these bacteria are influenced by what is called our natural resistance—by the circulating antibodies we have in our blood and by the ability of our white cells to destroy foreign invaders. This resistance, in turn, is related to our emotions and to the general state of our health. And that is why some women who have not had vaginitis for long periods of time will suddenly develop problems. Their resistance has been lowered, and the bacteria which have been there all along begin to multiply.

We should think of vaginitis in much the same way that we think of a sore throat, because the vagina and the mouth are very similar in all their reactions. Just as a throat culture may show the same bacteria to be present whether we have a sore throat or not, a vaginal culture can show bacteria even when a woman is not having symptoms. It is her resistance that will determine whether or not these bacteria are virile enough or present in large enough quantities to make her sick.

There are also similarities between a vaginal discharge and a runny nose. When we have a severe cold, the body is trying to flush out the infection by irrigating the nose. If a woman has a heavy vaginal discharge, this is nature's way of irrigating the vagina. The fluids are pouring out in an effort to dilute the irritants and cure the infection.

What are some common vaginal infections?

One common infection that produces a heavy, foul-smelling discharge is caused by a protozoan known as Trichomonas. The trichomonad is a one-celled animal. When viewed under the microscope, it displays small eyes and projections. In various forms, the trichomonad can live in all types of mammals and birds. It often resides in a woman's vagina without causing any difficulty whatsoever until circumstances change her resistance or the numbers and types of bacteria in her vagina. Trichomonads then begin to multiply and cause a vaginal discharge that is frothy in texture and may be yellowish, greenish, or grayish in appearance.

A few trichomonads are often present in the vagina of women without symptoms. I remember one woman who illustrated the point quite well. This patient, who was postmenopausal, was having some difficulty with irritation of the vagina because of lack of estrogen. I put her on estrogenic therapy and she developed a severe trichomoniasis infection. The protozoans had apparently been in her vagina for a long period of time, but as we changed the chemistry of her vagina with the estrogen, the situation became favorable for the trichomonads to grow. We treated the infection, her body chemistry apparently adjusted, and she didn't have any more difficulty.

What is the treatment for trichomoniasis?

We are fortunate to have an oral medication specifically designed to attack this particular protozoan. It is called Flagyl and it is safe to use.

What are some other common vaginal infections?

Another common infection which produces intense inflammation and severe itching is caused by a yeast known as Candida albicans. Yeast is something that the human race has lived with for so many years, and the majority of people are reasonably resistant to it. So Candida is also found in the vagina of many women who do not have symptoms until some type of physical or emotional stress changes the body chemistry and allows the yeast to grow.

The most common instigator of a yeast infection is antibiotics. It doesn't matter what kind. Any antibiotic will enter the bloodstream and interfere with the bacteria in the vagina that maintain the protective acid environment. It is this acid environment which makes it difficult for other, abnormal bacteria to survive. So women who have recurring bouts of vaginal infection each time they are taking an antibiotic should tell their physician, because medication is available to counteract this problem.

Women who have diabetes may also have problems with their immunity to Candida. And pregnancy can be still another time when problems develop. During pregnancy the vagina tends to be more alkaline, and the woman's resistance tends to be lower, probably so that she will not reject the fetus growing inside her.

Finally, oral contraceptives can alter the acidity of the vagina and its resistance. Any discomfort should be reported to the gynecologist because yeast infections generally can be quickly and adequately treated with a number of medications that are presently available.

What about bacterial infections?

One of the major bacterial offenders is called Hemophilus vaginalis. These bacteria may also be present in the vagina without symptoms until there is a change in the woman's resistance which allows growth or colonization. That's when the vagina begins to produce a secretion in an effort to wash out the offenders, and the vulva becomes irritated with this secretion, which contains the breakdown products of the infection. Bacterial infections can be treated with antibiotics or sulfa creams. In addition, we have recently found that Hemophilus infections of the vagina respond to Flagyl, the same drug used for the treatment of Trichomonas.

What are some common causes of allergic vaginitis?

Some of the greatest offenders right now are the various flavored douches that are a favorite with young people. These douches are used so that when the man practices oral sex he can taste the fruity flavor.

Vaginal sprays and deodorants can also cause allergic reactions and irritations, as can certain soaps and detergents. Additional problems may be caused by nylon-type underclothes, which do not absorb the moisture on the vulva and which increase the body heat, setting the stage for any bacteria that are present to multiply and grow in the lower part of the vagina and on the vulva.

Women who are having this difficulty should switch to cotton underclothes. In fact, they should stop wearing any underclothes at all around the house and should discontinue the use of any irritating soaps or vaginal sprays.

Are there other things a woman can do to help her vaginitis?

If the woman has a small amount of irritation on the inside of her vulva, or vaginal lips, she can try a simple, home remedy mini-douche. She can buy a small, inexpensive douche bag and put in one teaspoon of vinegar with one six-ounce glass of water. She can douche with this three times a day and at bedtime and increase the acidity of the vagina so that her natural resistance returns and the irritation goes away. This is like gargling with hot salt water, which is the proper treatment for a minor sore throat.

Of course, if the problem gets no better the woman needs to see a physician, and he must examine the vaginal discharge under the microscope. The physician should not treat vaginitis merely by writing a prescription. He must take a sample of the discharge and study it under the microscope. It's impossible to make a correct diagnosis any other way.

Can the doctor actually see what is causing the infection?

Not always. Although he is able to see Trichomonas or yeast, there are other times he can only see signs or "clue cells" of an infectious agent. Here the gynecologist makes his diagnosis by exclusion. He hasn't found Trichomonas or yeast, but he knows the woman is infected because she has symptoms. So he treats this nonspecific infection, often by using a sulfa cream, which is applied in the vagina and which reduces the number of bacteria so that the body regains its balance and corrects its problem. Here again, we are merely helping the body to help itself.

If a woman has recurring bouts of nonspecific infection, and I know this from repeatedly examining her vaginal discharge under the microscope, I may suggest the use of boric acid. This is the simplest, cheapest, and most effective drug to treat recurrent vaginitis. The boric acid is placed in large gelatin capsules and used nightly in the vagina for seven days. Because of the acidity of the capsule, the vagina is put back in balance, and the bacterial infection generally disappears.

If a woman has a vaginal infection, must she abstain from sexual intercourse?

It is true that certain types of infection, such as trichomoniasis, can be transferred back and forth between sexual partners. On the other hand, trichomonads will not generally live in a man's body unless he is having problems with his own resistance. Or he may retain the trichomonads in a harmless state until a later date when his resistance becomes lowered, and he develops symptoms in his prostate or urethra. Then he can transfer it back to the woman if her resistance is down.

If the diagnosis of trichomoniasis is correctly made, the proper medication will kill the protozoans in seven days. Until then I would recommend abstaining from sex.

Yeast infection can also be transmitted sexually, although here again the partner's resistance must be lowered to the point where the yeast can grow. You can put yeast on a man's penis, but if he has good resistance, it doesn't bother him. On the other hand, yeast does tend to grow under the foreskin of the uncircumsized penis. So if a woman who has a long-term relationship with an uncircumsized male has repeated bouts of yeast infection, and this infection has been carefully diagnosed, this may be good reason for the male to be circumsized, provided he, too, is found to have the infection and they are obviously transferring it back and forth.

Please discuss how emotional upsets can cause vaginitis.

If a woman has a heavy amount of vaginal secretion that is clear in color and does not cause itching, and her doctor finds no Trichomonas, no yeast, and no clue cells, then he will know that this problem is most likely caused by emotional factors.

The principle here is precisely the same as when a person has an ulcer. Just as the ulcer victim is putting out an excessive amount of gastric juice when he is under stress, this woman is putting out increased amounts of vaginal secretion—not from the uterus but from the cervix and from the secretory cells in the walls of the vagina.

I once had a twenty-two-year-old, virginal patient who had been treated by other physicians for a condition which had been diagnosed as yeast infection. Over a period of three years, she had visited five different physicians, who had prescribed various medications.

When I examined her vulva, there was no real evidence of irritation or itching. There was a moderate amount of vaginal secretion, but this was very clear and appeared quite normal. When I examined the secretion under the microscope, there was no yeast, no Trichomonas, and no clue cells. It was evident that the secretion was perfectly normal.

I discussed my findings with the patient and then proceeded to talk about some of the emotional factors in her life. She was a very obsessive, tense individual who worked very intently at her job. Peer acceptance was extremely important, and she was greatly concerned whenever she felt she had made someone angry or upset. In the course of our discussion we established that her vaginal secretion was much less under situations of no stress, such as weekends, vacations and whenever she could find time for reading, which she enjoyed very much.

At my suggestion this patient began using cornstarch to prevent the irritation of her vagina. She switched to cotton panties and whenever possible went without them. She gave up pantyhose and went back to stockings. And by coming to understand that her emotional problems were aggravating the situation, the patient improved 75 percent. It was no longer necessary for her to use all those useless medications which had been prescribed previously.

Emotionally caused vaginitis can be difficult to treat, but as soon as the patient understands the real source of her problems, we are a long way toward correcting the situation.

How does not wearing underclothes help vaginitis?

Nature did not intend for people to wear underclothes, and women were not meant to keep their vulva wrapped up all day. Bacteria thrive in a warm, moist climate, so adequate air circulation keeps the lips of the vagina dry and deprives bacteria of the moisture they need to grow.

Why are many older women plagued with vaginitis and irritation of the vulva?

Postmenopausal vaginitis is due to the fact that the lining of the vagina, which is actually made of skin similar to the skin on the palm of the hand, becomes very thin because of lack of estrogen. When this happens, the bacteria which are present can colonize and grow, and this causes pain and discomfort.

The postmenopausal vagina can be treated very successfully with a small amount of cream containing estrogen.

It is important to note, however, that women who have a vulva with very thin skin and reddish spots should see a physician. Many times this is a dermatologic condition which can be treated with the male hormone, testosterone, in a petroleum jelly. The testosterone makes the skin much firmer and reduces the irritation. This then stops the scratch-itch syndrome which so many women develop when they have irritation of the vulva. But this is not something a woman can treat by herself. It's important that she be seen by a physician and preferable that he perform a biopsy of certain areas of the vulva to rule out cancer and confirm his diagnosis.

Another problem involves raised or whitish sores on the vulva. These sores or lesions, known as leukoplakia, may on rare occasions be associated with cancer and must be biopsied by a physician. Once the diagnosis is made, this problem can be treated very successfully with cortisone.

What causes vaginal odor?

This is an area of much misinformation. The inside of the vagina doesn't smell bad. It is the bacteria growing on the moist vulva which produce the body odor that women smell. This is similar to the situation in which bacteria grow and cause odor in the armpit.

Women who think they have an odor or who have a constantly moist and irritated vulva should dry themselves thoroughly after bathing or going to the bathroom. They, too, should liberally apply cornstarch to the vulva so that the bacteria have no moisture in which to grow. I think I have helped more women with this simple technique than with any other measure. Occasionally a Hemophilus infection inside the vagina causes an odor.

We have heard a great deal about vaginal abnormalities in daughters of women who took the drug DES when they were pregnant. Exactly what was the cause of the problems here?

The drug diethylstilbestrol (DES) was widely prescribed in the late forties and fifties to prevent miscarriage. Some of the female off-spring of women who took this drug during the first eighteen weeks of pregnancy do have structural abnormalities in the vagina, in the mouth of the womb, and in the womb itself. It is also true that a very small—and I must emphasize a very, very small—group of these girls develop an extremely rare cancer that is related to their mother's having taken DES. Only about two hundred cases of cancer have been found among the several million offspring of women who took DES. This medication also has caused some structural changes among males, but no cancer.

Most of the problems associated with DES involve defects in the skin of the vagina, up around the mouth of the womb. These daughters may also have excessive numbers of secretion-producing cells in their vagina and on their cervix.

So if a woman knows that she took stilbestrol, it is important for her daughter to be examined around the time she begins to have menstrual periods so that if she does have vaginal irregularities they can be treated. Of course, if the girl has irregular bleeding prior to menstruation she should also see a doctor. The rare cancers that have occurred were found most frequently among girls who were not yet menstruating but had irregular bleeding.

At the present time we believe that if these girls do not have signs of cancer by the time they begin menstruating, they will not develop it.

How should these girls be examined?

The first thing they should have is a digital examination in which the gynecologist tries to pass his fingers along the entire area of the vagina. In this way he may be able to feel any abnormality (or adenosis) even if he is unable to see it. Of course, if he feels any abnormalities, they should be biopsied.

Many gynecologists also feel that the colposcope should be used. The colposcope is a binocular type of optical instrument that has a light source and can magnify the skin of the vagina about ten times. This apparatus enables the physician to inspect the cells of the vagina in more detail and if necessary can enable him to take a small biopsy of sample cells for further diagnosis.

Finally we take Pap smears, not only of the cervix but of the vagina, and once this is done the examination is as thorough as we can make it. We suggest that the patient come back for a regular examination every six months, and I might also suggest that she insert boric acid capsules about three times a week if there are abnormal changes in the vagina and on the cervix. This will keep the vagina slightly acid so the skin will be stimulated to grow in areas where it is deficient.

Some women are bothered by chronic cysts of the vagina or cervix. What should they know about these?

They should know that most of these cysts require no treatment whatsoever, while others must be opened and drained.

Cysts on the cervix, known as Nabothian cysts, are caused by mucus which has been trapped behind a small, closed gland. These cysts may reach the size of a fingernail, but they generally do not need to be drained or treated.

Cysts which occur on the walls of the vagina are known as Gartner's duct cysts and are filled with a clear fluid. Although these cysts may reach the size of a hen's egg, they do not need to be removed either, unless they cause pain during intercourse or obstruction during childbirth, both very rare.

One type of cyst which may require treatment, however, results from blockage of the pea-sized glands just inside the vaginal opening. These Bartholin's glands, as they are called, now serve no purpose whatsoever. At one time the odor from these glands may have identified those women who were in their fertile period. These Bartholin's glands occasionally form cysts which may eventually become abscessed and extremely painful. Then the physician must open and drain the cyst, a procedure he can usually perform in his office using local anesthesia.

BLADDER DISORDERS

Why are women more prone to bladder problems than men?

The female urethra (the tube which carries urine from the bladder) is located just above the opening of the vagina. The urethra is short in length and can be easily contaminated by vaginal bacteria. The male urethra, on the other hand, is quite long, so that bacteria have more difficulty reaching the bladder.

Another problem for the female involves childbirth, which often stretches and damages the pelvic muscles that support the urethra and the bladder. This damage may cause the woman to have less control over the elimination of her urine.

What causes the bladder problem known as cystitis?

Cystitis is an inflammation of the bladder most often caused by bacteria which are transferred from the rectum to the vagina and then to the urethra. A woman may have developed resistance to these bacteria in her rectum and vagina, but until she gains a similar resistance in her bladder, symptoms occur.

What are these symptoms?
The patient feels as if she has to urinate frequently because the bladder has become irritated in its effort to rid itself of bacteria. To make matters worse, the urination is often accompanied by a severe burning sensation and occasionally by bleeding. This is because the bladder responds to the invasion of the bacteria by increasing its blood supply.

What causes "honeymoon cystitis"?
A woman who has never had intercourse has never had her vaginal bacteria massaged into her urethra by the thrusting of the penis. So the bacteria multiply and grow in a urethra which has already suffered some minor injury during the act of intercourse.

That is why it is my usual practice to give a woman a prescription for sulfa drugs when I see her for a premarital examination, particularly if she has not been having regular intercourse. One day I offered such a prescription to a young patient but she refused, explaining that she had had intercourse frequently and didn't expect any problems. I tried to insist that she might have intercourse even more frequently and more vigorously during her honeymoon, but she preferred not to take any drugs. This young lady and her new husband went to Las Vegas and apparently had a really great time. But sure enough, by having intercourse three or four times a day she contracted a rip-roaring case of honeymoon cystitis. It took her more than twenty-four hours to locate a physician and obtain the prescription I had tried to send with her.

How is cystitis treated?
The physician should take a specimen of the urine in order to culture and identify the bacteria. Sulfa drugs are usually effective, and then the patient may never have another attack because the majority of women develop resistance to the bacteria introduced into their bladder during intercourse.

Occasionally a woman may have an especially short urethra, which makes it easier for vaginal bacteria to gain entrance to her bladder, and if her defense mechanisms are weakened, she will suffer repeated bouts of cystitis. Any woman who has chronic urinary-tract infection should be placed on antibiotics for a considerable period of time—

two or three weeks. Cultures should also be taken of her urine to be sure that the infection has not progressed into her kidneys, where it can become life-threatening.

Are there ways a woman can help herself with chronic cystitis?

Because the infection in her bladder originally comes from her rectum, the woman should cleanse properly after each bowel movement. She should wipe from front to back in order not to transfer excessive bacteria from the rectum into her vagina or urethra.

If she continues to suffer attacks, she might also try this procedure: following intercourse she should immediately urinate in order to wash out the bacteria which have been put into the urethra by the thrusting penis. Then she should drink two glasses of water, which will cause her to void once again in several hours; this will flush out her bladder a second time. If this simple technique is not effective, her physician can prescribe appropriate medication to be taken after intercourse.

It is particularly important during an acute attack of cystitis, and probably for the first week afterward, that the patient not drink alcoholic beverages. Alcohol interferes with the work of the white cells in resisting the disease and allows the bacteria to grow more readily in the urine.

I remember one patient who was just getting over a severe bout of cystitis when she was taken out to a very fine restaurant for dinner, and her escort ordered an excellent bottle of wine. Although I had warned the patient that she should not drink any alcohol for at least two weeks after she discontinued her medication, she succumbed to temptation. Within two days, she had a severe recurrence of her cystitis, and I finally had to send her to a urologist for some complex tests and treatments. She told me that was the most expensive bottle of wine she ever drank.

Why do some women lose urine when they cough or sneeze?

Stress incontinence, as this condition is called, occurs when there has been some breakdown in the mechanism by which a woman holds her urine. If the tissues surrounding the urethra have been weakened because of aging, a reduction in hormones, or the trauma of childbirth, the junction between the urethra and the bladder does not remain closed, and urine is lost involuntarily when there is the pressure of coughing, sneezing, or awkward movements. If sufficiently severe, this type of stress incontinence can be corrected by very special surgery.

If the problem is not severe, exercises may help the patient develop better control. The woman should practice voiding, then stopping, then voiding, then stopping, until she improves her muscle tone.

She can also practice contracting her vaginal muscles. A woman who does not know how to accomplish this can insert several fingers into her vagina and learn, by trial and error, to tighten those muscles which she feels are squeezing her fingers.

This problem of stress incontinence is not to be confused with an entirely different problem, known as "urge incontinence," which is caused by an infection of the neck of the bladder. Here the bladder recognizes that it is infected and attempts to squeeze out the irritant material. The patient is unable to control the urethra, and urine is lost. The treatment for urge incontinence should be provided by a competent urologist.

Is it true that "nerves" can cause a woman to urinate frequently?

Because a bladder can tense up under emotional stress just like any other area of the body, emotional tension can indeed cause a woman to urinate frequently. This problem is often helped simply by having the gynecologist explain the situation so that the woman does not compound the tension by excessive worry. Occasionally the doctor may prescribe tranquilizers or other medication to counteract bladder spasms.

Regrettably, many unnecessary operations are performed because a distinction has not been made between a bladder which has some slight infection, a bladder which has an anatomical defect, and an unstable bladder which exhibits its symptoms when the woman is under emotional stress. Unfortunately some physicians do not take a thorough enough history and do not perform a complete examination when there is stress incontinence. This may result in unnecessary or even improperly performed operations.

How should the correct diagnosis be made?

I prefer to use the urethroscope, which is a very small telescopic instrument that has a light source and carbon dioxide flowing through it. The urethroscope can be passed into the bladder without any pain or discomfort and the physician can determine if there is any chronic inflammation of the bladder caused by an infection.

Then by looking at the junction between the urethra and bladder as the gas passes through, and by asking the patient to bear down, the physician can see whether the sphincter of the bladder closes properly. It should close down much like the diaphragm in a camera.

You can see it closing and getting smaller and smaller if the woman has no anatomical defect.

Through the use of the urethroscope, we also have the ability to graph the reaction of the bladder to carbon dioxide. The unstable, or nervous, bladder is characterized by irregular swings on this graph, telling us that these patients do not require an operation, but can be treated with certain medications.

11

FIBROID TUMORS, ENDOMETRIOSIS, AND OVARIAN CYSTS

FIBROID TUMORS

Everybody talks about fibroid tumors of the uterus, but nobody explains what they are.

A fibroid tumor is a mass of muscle wrapped in fibrous, or connective, tissue. Fibroids, which can occur anywhere in the body, seem to be related to aging and heredity. They tend to occur more frequently among black women and among women whose ancestors came from the Middle East and Mediterranean areas.

What causes fibroids?

We do not know why these cells develop and grow. Although the body recognizes them as being somewhat abnormal, the immune system wages no attack as it would on other disease. Instead the body envelops these muscle cells in a fibrous capsule so they remain attached to the uterine wall, distorting its size and shape.

Are fibroids dangerous?

Fibroids are rarely, if ever, malignant. Maybe one half of 1 percent will ever lead to cancer, and these tend to be in women who have had large, neglected fibroids for many years.

No one should have a hysterectomy for fear of cancer developing in fibroids unless the tumor is growing rapidly—even though some physicians do use this threat as a reason for removing the uterus. Even if a woman has four or five small fibroids and her uterus feels lumpy when she is examined by her gynecologist, it doesn't mean that the uterus is abnormal and must be removed. A woman who had a hysterectomy for a fibroid the size of a hen's egg was probably talked into an operation she did not need, or she really wanted to be sterilized and used the fibroid as an excuse.

I have had interesting conversations with Catholic physicians who, after they get a bit older, will admit that many of the hysterectomies they performed on their patients were not for disease but for sterilization. Since they were working in Catholic hospitals, where sterilizations are not permitted, they would indicate that the problem was fibroids.

Are fibroids dangerous during pregnancy?

A woman can have a successful pregnancy with fibroids of tremendous size, and it is wrong for a physician to tell her that she or her baby is in serious danger. It is rare for fibroids to cause a miscarriage, and I usually encourage a woman who has large fibroids to complete a pregnancy that is underway and then consider a hysterectomy at a later date if she has finished her childbearing.

This point is illustrated by a patient who was treated in my department. The patient was a thirty-year-old unmarried woman with large fibroids. She had wanted to have a child all of her adult life despite the fact that she was single, and she was very much supported in this desire by her family. She finally did conceive and came in to see us when she was supposedly eight weeks pregnant. Her womb had already expanded above her navel, and we could feel fairly large tumors on both sides of her abdomen. We already knew that the patient had fibroids, but her right ovary also seemed somewhat enlarged, and we had to be sure she did not have ovarian cancer.

We operated on this patient, knowing that she desperately wanted to keep the pregnancy, and what we found was extremely large fibroids.

In the process of exploring the abdomen, one of the fibroids broke away from the wall of the uterus, and it was necessary for us to give the patient three units of blood before we could get the uterus repaired. Since she did not have cancer, we did not disturb the pregnancy and closed the abdomen—even though she had these enormous fibroids which would give her a considerable amount of pain and discomfort. The fibroids were so large, in fact, that we actually had trouble closing the abdomen.

The patient had a terrible time during the remainder of her pregnancy. She had constant pain. She had to use ice caps on her abdomen, and we had to give her codeine at periodic intervals to relieve her discomfort. But she wanted to have the baby, and she had tremendous support from her family.

She became so large that she could hardly walk, and it became apparent that she was going to have twins. Despite the discomfort and pain, despite the necessity of being in the hospital five or six times, despite the necessity of extensive bed rest, she delivered her twins quite successfully. She had accomplished what she wanted to do.

When do fibroids require a hysterectomy?

There are several good reasons for removing a uterus enlarged by fibroid tumors. One is size alone, when the uterus becomes enlarged to the point where it is at least ten centimeters, or four inches, above the pubic bone. In this situation, there is a good possibility that there will later be bleeding and pain, and the enlarged uterus may eventually obstruct vital organs.

Another good reason for performing a hysterectomy is when a fibroid causes excessive bleeding. This happens when the tumor grows through the wall of the uterus into its lining, or when the blood supply of the fibroid creates extra bleeding during the menstrual process. In women over the age of thirty-five, however, irregular bleeding must always be considered a possible sign of cancer, so a D&C must first be performed to make an accurate diagnosis.

Still another legitimate reason for a hysterectomy is rapid growth of the fibroid. When cancer does occur, rare though it may be, it is generally associated with this symptom. So if a physician finds that a tumor has greatly increased in size during a six-month period, that may be a good reason for surgery.

Many women resist a hysterectomy because they associate the loss of their uterus with the loss of their femininity.

I am fully aware that the loss of reproductivity can be threatening to many women, but the argument that the uterus is an essential aspect of femininity is simply not true. The uterus has one single purpose: to carry and nourish the growing fetus. The uterus has no relationship whatsoever to a woman's sexuality or her ability to make love.

I realize, however, that just because *I* think it's foolish for a woman to grieve over a lost uterus doesn't mean that *she* thinks it's absurd. If she is having this particular problem, I try to understand, to talk about it and help her accept the situation

I am finding a growing cult against hysterectomies, probably the result of the feminist movement. A number of articles that adversely deal with the operation have been written in women's magazines, and I'm sure some of these articles are based on fact. Sometimes the operations are performed without truly informed consent. But women should understand that very few operations are a matter of life and death, and hysterectomies are sometimes performed to improve the patient's comfort and well-being. So patients who need the operation should not be misled. Why should they continue to suffer with bleeding problems when the quality of their lives can be improved?

"Hysterectomy" is not a bad word. It's an effective operation *if you really need it,* and many women tell me their life became much more pleasant after their operation.

I can remember one patient with such heavy bleeding from fibroid tumors that she used forty or fifty pads in one menstrual period. Occasionally she had to wear rubber pants so the blood wouldn't run through her clothes. This woman vehemently opposed hysterectomy because she had read that her vagina would be shortened and that her sexual desires would be lessened. In a last-ditch effort to control the profuse bleeding she went to a hypnotist. It was only when he could not help her that she consented to the operation.

A hysterectomy was performed through the vagina. The surgery took about thirty-five minutes, and the patient recovered beautifully. Later she was actually embarrassed about her previous reluctance, and now she explains to some of her friends who are undergoing the same operation that a hysterectomy is not a difficult thing. Her vagina has not been shortened, her sex life is better than ever, and she is relieved of the great burden which not only made her uncomfortable but prevented her from doing many of the things that made her life enjoyable.

But how can a woman protect herself from needless surgery?

By knowing the proper reasons to have a hysterectomy and by questioning her doctor carefully before she gives her consent. If a woman is having excessive bleeding, for instance, it may have nothing at all to do with her fibroid tumors. She may have "dysfunctional bleeding," as we have discussed. Here the problem may be caused by emotional stress and hormonal imbalance. In this case the bleeding might be helped simply by placing the woman on oral contraceptives for a few months.

If a woman has fibroids, she should make certain they are serious enough to require surgery because it is true that many unnecessary operations are performed on account of fibroids. I recall one patient who had a series of small harmless fibroids studded all over her uterus. There was no abnormal bleeding and the inside of her womb was perfectly normal in size and shape. When the surgeon removed her uterus, he showed it to the husband, who was delighted that this terrible-looking thing had been removed. True, the uterus did not look particularly good, but it certainly was functional, and none of the criteria for hysterectomy were present.

Vaginitis is another absolutely wrong reason for having a hysterectomy. As we have already noted, vaginitis can be treated with much simpler methods.

So my advice to women is to become informed, to have really thoughtful discussions with their doctor, and to ask themselves, "Must I really have this operation? What does it involve? And what are my alternatives?"

Any woman who has questions or doubts concerning her need for an operation should seek a second opinion or delay her decision if cancer is not involved. A hysterectomy is rarely an emergency operation. It's important that a woman take her time and be satisfied with her decision.

We have been hearing a great deal about "ghost surgery." How can a woman be sure that her own physician and not an assistant or resident performs her operation?

The only way to be certain is to ask him whether he intends to perform the entire operation himself. Even if he says yes, the patient must understand, however, that it is impossible for a surgeon to perform every detail of a major operation alone. He must have help. A trained assistant or resident allows the surgeon to operate quickly, smoothly, and effectively. And the resident may indeed perform part of the operation, particularly when the structures are nearer to him than to the surgeon. Time is of the essence in surgery, and any assistance which safely speeds up the course of the procedure is beneficial to the patient.

What's more, having a resident participate in the surgery improves the quality of postoperative care because the resident, who provides much of this care, is more aware of the details and possible complications of the operation.

Does a hysterectomy bring on menopause?

No, because the ovaries are not removed. A hysterectomy involves only the removal of the uterus. A hysterectomy *may*, however, bring on menopause several years earlier than would have occurred otherwise since some of the blood supply to the ovaries is reduced by the operation.

What, then, is meant by surgical menopause?

A surgical menopause occurs when there has been removal of *both* ovaries in an operation known as oophorectomy. (A surgical menopause will not occur if only one ovary has been removed.) Sometimes the ovaries are removed because they are diseased or cancerous or the woman has endometriosis. Other times the ovaries are removed in conjunction with a hysterectomy as a preventive measure.

However, if a woman is already menopausal, if she has already stopped menstruating, and she is having a hysterectomy for fibroids or some other condition, I believe her ovaries should be removed at the same time, so they won't later become a source of ovarian cancer, which can be a particularly lethal problem. In this case we are not changing the hormonal condition of the patient, who is already menopausal; we are merely surgically removing her ovaries.

We have not really improved our cure rate of ovarian carcinoma in the last twenty years because we have no good techniques for early diagnosis. We can't take a Pap smear of the ovary, and the cancer develops very slowly, as it does in the breast. By the time we are able to feel it, the malignancy has often proceeded to the point where it is incurable. So in women who are already menopausal, we always remove the ovaries during a hysterectomy—provided that the patient gives her consent.

But isn't surgical menopause more severe than natural menopause?

To some degree, it may be—especially in younger women. In younger women who have had their ovaries removed, the production of estrogen has suddenly been cut off, and the reproductive hormones in the brain don't understand this. These hormones keep trying to make the missing ovaries do their work. Estrogen replacement therapy must be used to reduce, or even eliminate, symptoms of low estrogen level. Older women may not need estrogen replacement because their adrenal glands may already be taking up the slack. The physician can determine this by his examination of the vagina and discussing the patient's symptoms.

It has been my experience that women below the age of forty-five need hormonal replacement after losing their ovaries. I feel that if the physician refuses to provide this treatment, the woman should seek another doctor. That may seem a bit rough on the gynecologist, but I believe it's necessary, especially since there is no chance of the estrogen's causing uterine cancer since the uterus has been removed.

If a woman under the age of forty-five is having a hysterectomy, why should her healthy ovaries be removed to prevent a cancer that may never occur? This seems too radical a procedure.

I agree, and this question is a source of controversy among many physicians. In her book *The Petticoat Surgeon*, Dr. Bertha van Hoosen observed that male surgeons seldom found an ovary good enough to keep or a testicle quite bad enough to take out.

I have to admit that we see lots of ovaries but very few testes in pathology museums. The fact is that years ago many surgeons did not fully understand gynecologic disease, and they might have removed ovaries unnecessarily.

I don't like to remove an ovary unless I feel that I must. My general rule is that I will remove both ovaries in women over forty-five because the ovaries will probably not function much longer anyway, and we can reduce the possibility of later cancer. Prior to that age, I remove only diseased ovaries, and I place the patient on estrogen therapy.

What will it do to a woman's sex life if her ovaries are removed?

The principles of treatment for the surgical menopause are the same as for the normal menopause. If the woman's sex life was good before the operation, it's going to continue to be good. Just because she can no longer ovulate or conceive does not mean she cannot enjoy sex and have a good strong orgasm. Of course, as we have said, younger women whose ovaries have been removed should take estrogen replacement so they don't have a reduction of their vaginal secretions or dryness of the vagina and vulva.

What are the main dangers of a hysterectomy?

The major danger of any operative procedure involves anesthesia. This danger is extraordinarily small and depends upon the age as well as medical and surgical problems of the patient. If the patient has had no previous medical problems and the anesthesia is being administered by a competent anesthesiologist or nurse anesthetist in an accredited hospital, the risk is minimal. Most problems that do arise are due to tracheal obstruction and the inability of the patient to breathe. That is why it is extremely important that all patients undergoing general anesthesia have a special hollow tube placed down their trachea, ensuring that the passageway will remain open.

In spinal anesthesia there is always the danger of injury to the spinal cord, but again this is a very small risk, maybe one in five thousand cases. If a patient has a competent anesthesiologist, this problem will be kept at an absolute minimum.

Possibly a more common surgical danger involves the development of pneumonia. This problem occurs in patients who have not had proper ventilation of the lungs while they were under anesthesia and who have not coughed and breathed deeply following the operation. This problem, of course, can be diagnosed quickly and treated with antibiotics.

There are other potential complications associated with the surgery itself. The most frequent is postoperative infection. When the uterus is removed through the vagina or abdomen, the bacteria normally present in the vagina are introduced into the abdominal cavity, which has limited resistance to these bacteria. The development of an abdominal infection will depend upon the strength or virulence of the bacteria, the immune response of the patient, and the length and difficulty of the operation.

The most frequent surgical injury during gynecologic surgery is to the large or small bowel. It is evident in figure 7 that the rectum is directly behind the uterus and the small bowel surrounds the pelvic structures. The bowel is most frequently injured when it becomes attached to the pelvic organs because of endometriosis, pelvic infection, or cancer. These injuries are generally easily repaired.

The second most frequently injured structure is the bladder; fortunately, this occurs rarely. The bladder must actually be pushed off the uterus to the upper part of the vagina. It is during this surgical maneuver that it may be injured. The injury occurs most often when there is cancer, infection in the pelvis, endometriosis, poor blood supply (as in older women), or previous pelvic operations, including cesarean section.

Fortunately, the most rare injury to the pelvic organs during gynecologic surgery, since it is the most difficult to repair, is an injury to a ureter, the small tube that brings urine from the kidney to the bladder. This tube runs beneath the vessels of the ovary and the uterus and enters the bladder less than one inch from the lower part of the uterus. It is most frequently injured when there is a large ovarian cyst, a pelvic infection, large fibroids on the side of the uterus, cancer, or endometriosis.

The possibility of pelvic infection and injury to these structures must be considered by any woman contemplating gynecologic surgery. The injuries may be due to an error by the surgeon, but they are usually related to the difficulty and seriousness of the operation.

Are there different types of hysterectomies?

Yes, there are. There are partial and total hysterectomies, both of which may be performed through the abdomen or the vagina. Then there are radical hysterectomies, which are always performed through the abdomen.

What are the differences between partial, total, and radical hysterectomies?

A partial hysterectomy involves removal of only the main portion

FIGURE 7. THE CLOSENESS OF THE UTERUS TO STRUCTURES WHICH MAY BE INJURED DURING GYNECOLOGIC SURGERY

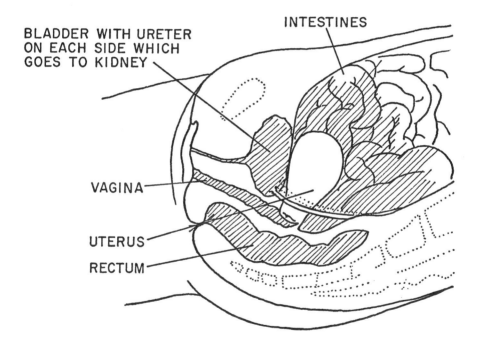

INTESTINES

BLADDER WITH URETER
ON EACH SIDE WHICH
GOES TO KIDNEY

VAGINA

UTERUS

RECTUM

VARIOUS GYNECOLOGIC OPERATIONS

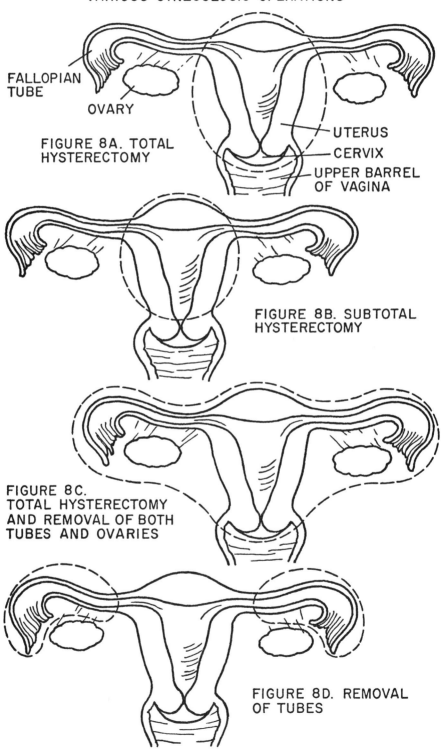

FALLOPIAN
TUBE

OVARY

UTERUS

CERVIX

UPPER BARREL
OF VAGINA

FIGURE 8A. TOTAL
HYSTERECTOMY

FIGURE 8B. SUBTOTAL
HYSTERECTOMY

FIGURE 8C.
TOTAL HYSTERECTOMY
AND REMOVAL OF BOTH
TUBES AND OVARIES

FIGURE 8D. REMOVAL
OF TUBES

of the uterus. The cervix, fallopian tubes, and ovaries are left intact. This operation is sometimes performed on patients with noncancerous pelvic disease, such as endometriosis, or extensive pelvic infection which makes it difficult to remove the uterus and cervix in their entirety, and the bulk of the disease lies in the removable portion.

A total hysterectomy involves removal of the cervix and the uterus but not the tubes or ovaries. In both operations, there is no change in a woman's hormones. She will no longer menstruate, but the ovaries are not removed. They will continue to produce estrogen, so the woman will not go through a surgical menopause. When the tubes and ovaries are also removed, the operation is called a total hysterectomy with bilateral salpingo-oophorectomy.

Next comes the radical hysterectomy, which is performed only for cancer. This surgery involves removal of the uterus, the cervix and adjacent tissues. We also remove the upper half of the vagina, the ovaries, fallopian tubes, the abdominal lymph nodes, and other areas where the cancer is likely to spread. This operation requires considerable skill and must be performed by a surgeon who has had special training.

Please compare vaginal versus abdominal hysterectomies. Who should have which?

The vaginal hysterectomy, in which the womb or uterus is removed through the vagina, is always preferred to opening the abdomen, provided there are no complicating factors. The vaginal hysterectomy takes about half the time and causes about half the pain because the abdominal skin and muscles have not been cut and the abdominal cavity has not been invaded, except for a short period of time.

The woman recovers much more rapidly because the body does not have to mend the layers of the abdominal wall. She will also have fewer problems with nausea and bowel discomfort. The vaginal hysterectomy is very safe when antibiotics are used to prevent infection and when the surgeon is skillful. Of course, another advantage is the fact that there is no abdominal scar.

I once had a patient who was a widow and very anxious not to have a scar, but her previous physician would not perform a vaginal hysterectomy because she had fibroids. These fibroids were not very large, and I performed the operation via the vaginal route. I recently saw this woman; she has now remarried and is very happy that she had her uterus removed in this fashion. So patients should never hesitate to discuss their preferences regarding incisions with their physicians.

However, if the patient has major problems with her ovaries or fallopian tubes or if there has been extensive infection or disease, the physician will need complete and full vision to operate safely, and he will therefore need to open the abdomen.

In general, no cancers of the pelvis should be treated by vaginal hysterectomy because the physician must inspect the abdomen carefully or must perform washings of the abdominal cavity for abnormal cells.

If a woman has very large fibroids, they are also difficult to remove safely through the vagina unless the surgeon is very skillful and can remove the fibroids one at a time before removing the entire uterus.

If they must have an abdominal hysterectomy, most women would prefer to have a horizontal incision for cosmetic reasons. When is this possible?

If a surgeon is performing a simple abdominal hysterectomy, if the uterus is not too large, and if there is not extensive pelvic disease, then a transverse, or horizontal, incision can be made. This incision (sometimes known as the bikini cut) is cosmetically preferable although it takes the surgeon longer to do the procedure and he really has less room in which to work unless he cuts some of the abdominal muscles.

The longitudinal, or vertical, incision gives the surgeon the best working area and allows him to explore the pelvis more completely. This incision can also be extended as high as needed if other problems are encountered.

How much pain should a woman expect following a hysterectomy?

There will be a considerable amount of discomfort during the first thirty-six hours following surgery. There will be pain in the incision and in the areas where the uterus or the tubes and ovaries have been removed. There may well be some nausea and vomiting, and there may be some intestinal cramps due to a temporary reduction in the function of the bowel. Another minor discomfort involves the inability to void. A catheter may be necessary for the first day or two, and this is perfectly normal.

Most patients require the use of some narcotics in the first few days after surgery, and it is important that these narcotics be used before the pain becomes unbearable. This early use of pain medication will not only make the first days of recuperation more comfortable, but will actually lead to less use of narcotics later in the recuperation period.

How much hospitalization is required following a hysterectomy?
Generally about one week.

Please describe the dos and don'ts of a proper recuperation.
Individual patients vary in their recuperative powers, so it is impossible to offer specific advice. In general, the first two weeks after hospitalization, a woman should behave as if she were still in the hospital. She should have no responsibility for preparing meals or cleaning the house. She should spend the majority of her time lounging in bed or on a sofa.

The third week she can begin to increase her activity somewhat. She can now leave the house for a brief visit, a movie, or a trip to a nearby restaurant for a relaxed dinner. But she should still remain careful not to overdo it because she will find that her strength is not yet back to normal.

The fourth week following the operation, the patient can begin to resume many of her old activities. She can begin to drive her automobile for short periods of time, and if she has had a vaginal hysterectomy she can even resume some minor exercises. If she has had an abdominal hysterectomy, however, this is usually not possible until after the fifth week.

When can a woman resume intercourse?
Usually not until six weeks following surgery, to ensure that the vaginal incision has healed and the thrusting of the penis will not interfere with the healing process. When sexual relations are first resumed, it is recommended to proceed carefully.

What do a woman's insides look like after a hysterectomy?
When the uterus is removed from the abdomen, the intestines fill the gap, just as they fill the male pelvis, which never had a uterus.

For women who truly oppose a hysterectomy, are there alternatives? Why can't a noncancerous or benign tumor, such as a fibroid, be removed with the uterus left intact?
Sometimes it can. This operation, known as a myomectomy, is most often performed on women who have not completed their childbearing activities and who feel they may later want to become pregnant. When the surgeon removes several fibroids, however, the uterus may be left scarred—often to the point where it might be more difficult to become pregnant and delivery must be by section since the damaged uterus might actually rupture during vaginal delivery.

So it is preferable to leave the fibroids alone until the patient has had as many children as she desires. The decision can then be made concerning a hysterectomy.

Although I understand the attitude about retaining the uterus if possible, in my opinion it is not advisable to perform multiple myomectomies and leave in a uterus which is not only useless but may later be associated with menstrual problems.

What's more, if the patient has the tendency to develop fibroid tumors, they will probably come back.

ENDOMETRIOSIS

What is endometriosis?

Endometriosis occurs when cells from the uterine lining, or endometrium, begin to grow outside the womb. These cells may attach themselves to the ovary, the bladder, or the rectum.

Endometriosis is a common disorder among women of childbearing age. We can often see or feel the first evidence of this disease in young women who are only seventeen or eighteen years old.

There are many theories about the cause of endometriosis. The most frequent explanation is that the uterus in these patients has a tendency to contract in the wrong direction at the time of menstruation, so that the menstrual blood backs up into the fallopian tubes instead of being pushed out through the vagina. This blood may contain live cells, which may grow on the pelvic structures. However, since they are normal cells, the endometriosis never turns to cancer. Endometriosis may also be congenital if some of the cells of the lining of the uterus have developed in the abdominal cavity rather than in the womb as is normal.

What are the symptoms of endometriosis?

The most frequent symptoms are infertility, menstrual cramps, pain on intercourse, and general abdominal discomfort. The degree of pain is usually related to the extent and degree of the endometriosis.

How does the gynecologist make his diagnosis?

When he performs an internal examination, the physician will determine the amount of pain present when he moves the cervix. He will also find that when endometriosis is present, the uterus and ovaries will not move as freely as they should. The physician may also be able to feel the endometrial growths on the pelvic ligaments. If there is any question concerning the diagnosis, he should look inside the abdomen with a laparoscope to make a definite diagnosis before he initiates treatment.

What if the endometriosis is extensive?

Then the patient will have chronic pain and a 35 percent chance of infertility.

What can be done to treat endometriosis?

Sometimes no treatment at all is necessary. But when it is, either an oral contraceptive, an injection of a progestin, or an oral medication which suppresses ovarian function can be very successful in preventing spread of the disease. These substances cause regression of the endometrium, so there are fewer cells to work their way into the abdominal cavity through the tubes, and the endometrial implants which are already present in the abdominal cavity are reduced in size and blood supply.

Although surgery sometimes becomes necessary, it is most important that a patient discuss all of the ramifications of the management of endometriosis with her physician. Sometimes a combination of medical treatment and surgery is necessary.

I remember one young woman, an extremely attractive debutante, who began to have very severe and painful menstrual periods by the time she was seventeen or eighteen years old. When this woman was married at the age of twenty-five, she found that intercourse was painful. It became evident during her examination that her left ovary was partly attached to the side of her pelvis, and she had small nodules of endometriosis on the other ovary. She was first treated medically with large doses of oral contraceptives, but this treatment was not effective. This patient was extremely desirous of becoming pregnant, so we performed a thorough examination of her husband and found he had normal fertility. Further testing on the patient herself uncovered no fertility problems other than the endometriosis, so a conservative operation was performed leaving her uterus. It was necessary to totally remove her left ovary along with small pieces of endometriosis on the right ovary. At the conclusion of surgery, this young woman was left with only one small piece of healthy ovarian tissue about the size of a fingernail. Fortunately, she became pregnant within three months following the operation and delivered a son who became her sole heir to a large fortune.

OVARIAN CYSTS

What causes the cysts that grow on the ovary?

During the reproductive years, the ovaries initiate cycles of ovulation and menstruation. These sometimes lead to the development of normal, or physiological, cysts. These cysts arise when the ovarian follicle which was supposed to release the ripened egg somehow does not do its job. Ovulation does not occur, and the follicle grows larger and becomes cystic. Also sometimes ovulation does occur but the follicle, which then becomes known as the corpus luteum, does not disappear, and becomes cystic.

In a woman of reproductive age, this does not necessarily require an operation, particularly if the cyst is not causing any pain or discomfort. These cysts will occur sometime during almost every woman's reproductive years, and they generally disappear spontaneously. If they do not disappear by themselves, the physician should first place the patient on oral contraceptives, which will suppress the follicle-stimulating hormone and the luteinizing hormone. Without this stimulation the cysts gradually decrease in size and disappear. Oral contraceptives generally allow us to avoid an operation.

Suppose the woman is already on the pill and she develops an ovarian cyst?

If a woman is already taking contraceptive pills, she is not ovulating and no follicles are being formed. Any enlargements which are present on the ovary, therefore, must be presumed to be abnormal until proven otherwise. The physician can use ultrasound and/or laparoscopy to assist him in making a diagnosis and determining the appropriate treatment.

Are there other types of ovarian cysts?

Another common type, known as a dermoid, consists of skin, oil, hair, and occasionally a tooth. These cysts, which are almost always benign, are somewhat solid and often rise high in the pelvis because the oil has less specific gravity than the water of the body. These cysts tend to twist more readily than other ovarian enlargements. They can frequently be diagnosed by an X-ray finding of a piece of rudimentary tooth.

Finally there are cysts that are difficult to diagnose. They may be benign and they may be malignant, and there is no real way to differentiate except by having a pathologist examine the tissue. If a woman has pain and discomfort in her abdomen and her physician finds a cyst that is four or five inches in diameter, he must first try oral contraceptives. Then if the cyst does not respond, he must perform exploratory surgery and remove the cyst, either alone or in conjunction with the ovary.

Occasionally girls will develop precocious puberty. A six- or seven-year-old youngster will begin to have menstruation and enlargement of her breasts, and the physician will find a cyst or tumor on the ovary. This is called a granulosa cell tumor and it is generally not malignant.

When these girls are operated on and the tumor is removed, their breasts return to normal size and their early menstruation ceases. They grow into normal adulthood and are able to have children.

Why do some women have excrutiating pain with ovarian cysts?

Severe pain is usually a sign of hemorrhage, rupture, or twisting. Surgery is required for all of these.

What causes ovarian cysts in women past menopause?

Unlike the woman who is still in her childbearing years, the menopausal woman has no good medical reason to have an ovarian cyst. If one is found, it must be considered cancerous until proven otherwise, and often it does turn out to be malignant. In such a patient, the necessary laboratory tests must be performed along with an immediate operation by a surgeon who is experienced in the treatment of ovarian cancer.

12

CANCER OF THE BREAST AND REPRODUCTIVE TRACT

If I could ask just one question with regard to cancer, it would have to be, "What can a woman do to avoid this dread disease?"

Before we can talk about preventing cancer, we must first understand its cause. Although we still have a lot to learn in this regard, we are beginning to fit together some bits and pieces of this great puzzle.

We know, for instance, that all living things—from plants to human beings—constantly produce abnormal cells. But these cells are recognized and destroyed by a healthy immune system before they grow out of hand. This immune system is what keeps us free from all disease, from cancer down to the common cold. It is only when the immune system becomes defective for any of a variety of reasons that some of these abnormal cells are not destroyed, and cancer is allowed to develop.

This often happens in the process of aging, and this is why older people are more vulnerable to cancer.

Are there ways to improve one's immunity to cancer?

Researchers are now seeking methods of bolstering the body's natural resistance to all kinds of disease, including cancer, and this is what the science of immunology is all about.

But for the average person with no sign of disease, the best rules for maintaining good immunity involve proper nutrition, adequate rest, sufficient exercise, and no more than a reasonable intake of alcohol and tobacco—the same rules that apply to maintaining general overall health.

We are also finding that a healthy mental outlook helps keep the immune system working efficiently. People who are not depressed or emotionally tense and upset tend to have fewer colds, and it just may be that they have fewer cancers.

But aren't there more specific ways of preventing cancer in the female organs?

Here again we need more research to understand what causes each particular kind of cancer before we can prevent it. We know, for instance, that cancer of the cervix appears to be related to early sexual intercourse and numerous partners. The younger a woman is when she begins having coitus and the more sexual partners she has, the more likely she is to develop this form of cancer.

We also know that cancer of the endometrium, or lining of the womb, is related to the excessive production of estrogen, a problem which tends to occur in women who ovulate and menstruate infrequently, so that their uterine lining grows and grows. We can sometimes reduce this problem with periodic injections of progesterone or with birth control pills.

If a woman has regular gynecologic examinations, her doctor can judge the extent of estrogen production by the texture of the vagina. If he observes an excess of estrogen production in the menopausal patient, he may want to take periodic biopsies of her uterus so that he will be able to spot early abnormalities that may be easily corrected. Menopausal women who are taking hormones should definitely have such an endometrial biopsy once a year. I should also mention that women who have diabetes or hypertension, women who are obese, and women who have never had children have a greater risk of acquiring cancer of the endometrium. This may be due to changes in the immune system.

When it comes to cancer of the vulva, we believe that personal hygiene plays a big role. When I was in Iran I was interested to learn that cancer of the vulva was almost nonexistent. One possible reason is that Iranian women remove their perineal hair because they do not consider it attractive. Their vulva is very clean, and cancer of the vulva is much less frequent. Also, most Iranian women do not have intercourse with various partners (although the Iranian younger generation is beginning to change in this regard), so these women are less exposed to cancer of the cervix and certain types of venereal diseases.

Is there anything a woman can do to prevent cancer of the breast?

We know that breast cancer is partly related to hereditary factors. We also think that women who nurse their children may acquire some protection. And the fact that Japanese and African women have very little breast cancer until they come to the United States has led us to believe there may be dietary or environmental influences. But these are not factors easily controlled, and so far we have no sure way to prevent breast cancer. The best we can offer is early detection through self-examination, regular checkups, and mammograms.

No female disease is more dreaded than cancer of the breast—not only because it can be lethal, but because a mastectomy can be so traumatic to a woman's self-esteem. What can a woman do to deal with such feelings?

Nobody wants to lose any part of her body. It is normal for there to be a period of grieving or mourning after an amputation of any sort, and there is no question that following a mastectomy a woman may mourn for her breast. There is a great sense of loss, and there is nothing wrong with her crying during this time and talking to her physician, her lover or husband, and her friends about how terrible it was for her to lose a part of her body.

There are women who mourn for their breast as they would mourn for the loss of a sibling or a child. And while grieving is important and therapeutic, it is best done by discussing one's emotions outwardly and venting the unhappiness and anxiety associated with the grief.

Doctors and patients must both accept the fact that there can be considerable rage in a patient who loses a breast—rage directed not only at the disease which caused this catastrophe but at the doctor who actually removed the breast. A woman should not be afraid to express this rage verbally, and the physician has the responsibility to allow the woman to vent her anger and grief because once these feelings are out of her system she will be more ready to move on with her life.

Following a mastectomy, many women feel that their femininity has been affected.

This feeling is understandable, but following a mastectomy a woman can continue to feel sexy and make just as fantastic love whether she has lost one or both of her breasts. These are not essential organs of her body. Nature intended breasts only for nursing an infant.

What if her husband or lover has always made a fetish out of her breasts?

Then he needs to be told, "You may be worried about my breast, but I'm worried about my life!" Breast cancer is the number one killer of premenopausal females in this country. One out of every fifteen American women will develop this disease during her lifetime, and 31,000 of these women will die each year. These statistics are uppermost in a doctor's mind when he is battling breast cancer, and women should explain these facts to their partners.

If a woman is faced with the possibility of losing a breast, it can be extremely difficult for her to voice these fears.

I realize there is no easy way to break this kind of news, but it must be done. The woman should simply say that she has a lump in her breast and she has to go into the hospital for a biopsy. The doctor hopes and believes the lump is benign, but there is always a possibility of cancer, in which case she may have to lose her breast. Most men who receive this news are extremely concerned about saving the life of the woman they love.

Let me tell you about a widow who had a lover of whom she was very fond. This woman developed cancer of the breast, so she went to the hospital, and her breast was removed. She developed a great fear that her lover would no longer care for her because she had lost her breast and was disfigured, and because she had had cancer, which in her mind was unclean. She worried and worried about this, and she finally came to talk with me.

She told me that although she continued to make love after the operation, she would never let her lover see her unclothed. So my advice was for her to take off her clothes and let her lover see her scar and touch it. I assured her this would make her feel more comfortable, and she would see that to a sweet, loving man the fact that she had only one breast would not matter.

The next time this couple made love, the woman took my advice. She asked her partner to touch her scar and to tell her what it meant to him. A few months later, she was back to see me, greatly relieved.

So we can't predict what losing a breast is going to mean to a man. Women have attributes which are interesting and exciting in addition to their breasts. Often it can be helpful for a woman who has had a mastectomy to be able to call on someone who has successfully gone through the same experience and can reassure her that she will not lose her femininity and all the very beautiful and subtle things that go with being a woman. There are groups of mastectomy patients who are willing to work with other women in this way, and I have found them to be extremely helpful. Women communicate with each other extremely well, and I think this approach can be quite beneficial.

If a woman has a family history of breast cancer, what are her odds of developing the disease?

A woman's chance of acquiring breast cancer increases two to eight times if her mother has had the disease. The risk grows even higher if her sister has had breast cancer. Such a woman should always inform her physician of her family history, because periodic mammograms are particularly important in her case. But even with a family history of cancer, the odds are still in a woman's favor. She is probably not going to develop the disease, although she is at higher risk than a woman who has no such history.

How are most breast cancers detected?

Most breast cancers are discovered by women themselves, and we have already talked about the importance of self-examination. Any breast lump, puckering of the skin, nipple discharge, or development of inversion of the nipple should be reported promptly to the woman's doctor.

Of course, some breast cancers are also detected during routine medical examinations, and still others are discovered through the use of mammography, thermography, and sonography.

But aren't mammograms dangerous? The controversy over radiation effects has many women frightened.

A mammogram, which is an X ray of the breast, is still the best diagnostic technique we have to detect early cancers before they can be felt during a regular examination. Today mammography is safer than ever with more modern equipment using less radiation. If a woman's breasts are consistently lumpy because her milk ducts are extensively clogged, her doctor can't examine her thoroughly by touch alone, and mammography is the best tool to do the job. Mammograms are also helpful in detecting early cancer in women who have a strong family history of breast cancer; for them the benefits far outweigh any small risk of radiation.

Mammograms, however, are not perfect. They do not detect all breast cancer and cannot be considered a clean bill of health. Just because the mammogram turns out normal does not mean that the patient does not need to continue her self-examinations.

Which women should and should not have routine mammograms?

Physicians generally feel that regular mammograms should be reserved for those women who are past the age of fifty because breast cancer occurs most frequently in this group. In these women there is no danger whatsoever of one mammogram per year causing cancer because the woman will not live long enough, or have enough mammograms, to suffer the effects of too much radiation. Over the age of fifty, the decreased amount of fat in the breast also allows a more accurate mammogram to be performed.

It is also a good idea for women in the thirty-five-to-fifty age bracket to have at least one mammogram in order to provide the physician with a record with which to compare later breast changes that may occur.

Women below thirty-five do not need a mammogram unless they have developed a suspicious lump, inversion of the nipple, nipple discharge, or chronic mastitis.

What is chronic mastitis?

Women often find small pebblelike lumps in their breasts. These pebbles are really a series of enlarged milk glands and the condition is called chronic cystic mastitis. It is caused by the stimulation of a woman's breast by estrogen and progesterone during the menstrual cycles. We must remember that a woman's breasts evolved to be used for nursing an infant for long periods of time, and when she is nursing, a woman does not have this hormonal stimulation. That is why women in primitive societies who are nursing infants for most of their reproductive lives do not develop chronic cystic mastitis.

Is cystic mastitis related to cancer?

Not per se, but there might be a cancerous lump amid the numerous little cysts, and this can be difficult to determine. If there is only a small number of cysts, or even one large solitary cyst, the doctor can attempt to draw out the fluid and send this material for diagnosis. But if a woman has extensive cystic mastitis, particularly if she is over the age of thirty-five or forty, it is difficult to determine which lumps are significant and which are not. In these cases, mammograms may be helpful.

What is the likelihood that a lump on the breast might be malignant?

The vast majority of lumps, possibly 80 percent, are not cancerous. The lump is usually just a cyst composed of fluid or a noncancerous tumor which can be removed by surgery. But all lumps must be reported immediately and carefully checked.

Which lumps are most suspicious?

A single lump in a woman past her teens may be suspect, although these are often noncancerous. The only way to be sure is to remove the lump or draw out its fluid and study the material under the microscope.

One harmless type of lump in young women is composed mostly of fibrous tissue. Such lumps are never malignant although the surgeon often removes them because the patient will worry excessively. These fibroadenomas are hard and distinct and movable because the skin is not attached to them.

You have mentioned breast thermography and sonography in connection with breast cancer detection. How do these techniques work?

Thermography, which measures the warmth of the breast without using X ray, is used to detect women at higher risk of developing breast cancer. Thermography is not as accurate as mammography in the actual diagnosis of cancer, but when a patient has a positive thermogram, her physician may want to watch her more closely. This does not necessarily mean she is going to develop breast cancer. About two thirds of those women who have a positive thermogram do not.

Sonography, otherwise known as ultrasound or sonar, uses high-frequency sound waves, far beyond the range of human hearing, to detect lumps or masses in the breast. Sonography, like thermography, uses no radiation, but, also like thermography, this technique is not nearly as accurate as mammography.

Once a lump is found in the breast, how does the doctor tell if it is cancerous?

The first thing the doctor tries to do is determine if the lump is a cyst. He does this by inserting a needle and attempting to draw out fluid in a procedure known as *aspiration.* If the laboratory tests determine that this fluid is noncancerous, there is generally no need for further treatment. It is not necessary for a woman to have surgery either for a biopsy or for removal of nonmalignant cysts, even though many surgeons do perform such procedures.

On the other hand, if the physician is unable to draw fluid from the tumor and it is composed of solid tissue, then the patient must undergo surgery for removal of the tumor so it can be studied under the microscope. While the patient is still under anesthesia in the operating room, a pathologist freezes the tumor, then slices a small piece, which he places on a slide and stains with a special dye.

Cancerous cells will absorb the dye differently from noncancerous ones. There will be a variation in size and shape so that the architectural pattern of the tissue will be destroyed. There may also be a clumping together of cancer cells. This is a very accurate method of diagnosing cancer of the breast.

How long does this test take?

Only about ten to twenty minutes.

What if the lump is found to be cancerous?

If the cancer is confined to the breast, that is, if it hasn't spread to other parts of the body, then surgery is the proper treatment.

In very early stages of the disease it may be possible to simply remove the tumor in a procedure known as lumpectomy. Then the breast and lymph nodes (which are the adjacent tissue) are given radiation therapy. There has been some experimental use of radiation therapy, and the preliminary five-year survival rates seem to be about 40 to 75 percent—not necessarily a high survival rate for small tumors. I must point out, however, that this work is very preliminary and we do not know the final outcome because when cancer is present in one part of the breast it may be present elsewhere in the breast. Thus the whole breast is best removed.

I must also point out that there are certain side effects with this radiation approach. The radiation tends to cause osteoporosis, or demineralization, of the ribs, rendering them more vulnerable to fracture. The treated breast may also shrink in size and turn brown, and there may be some scarring of the lung. So radiation therapy is not without its consequences.

Aren't there any other surgical options in breast cancer?

Although there are differences of opinion as to the extent of the surgery that is required, it is generally necessary to remove the entire breast because a doctor can never be sure of the extent of the disease. It is also important to remove the lymph nodes for two reasons: first, because this is where the cancer is most likely to spread, and second, by studying the nodes we can tell if this has already happened, in which case we will begin giving chemotherapy.

No longer do we remove any muscles from the chest wall. This used to be the most disfiguring part of this operation, and it also interfered with the strength and ability of the arm to move, particularly sideways. Women should defend themselves against this mutilating procedure by insisting that their doctor not remove the chest muscles. Removing these muscles has not been found to affect cure rates.

Why can't the mastectomy be performed several days after the biopsy to give the woman time to accept the idea of losing a breast?

Because there is no point in prolonging the decision. If cancer is present and it has not yet spread to other parts of the body, an operation is required as soon as possible.

Surely a few more days won't make much difference.

If the woman needs more time, she should probably not have the biopsy performed until she is ready to accept the diagnosis and have the necessary treatment. There is no point in subjecting her to a second dose of anesthesia unnecessarily. It is simply better medicine to proceed with the full operation, if that is what is needed.

Of course, if there is the slightest doubt in the doctor's mind or if the biopsy is inconclusive, it is necessary to perform a more complicated and time-consuming test known as a "permanent section." This test gives much more precise information, and until the results are in it is better to delay the mastectomy. We feel there is no danger in waiting for additional microscopic studies if there is the slightest chance of an error in diagnosis with the frozen section. But if there is no question it is unreasonable to have a second anesthetic.

How does breast cancer get out of control?

We have come to believe that all cancer spreads as a result of a breakdown in the immune system. The body does not recognize and destroy the abnormal cells, and they are allowed to spread through the lymphatic channels in the blood and lymph streams. Cancer of the breast most often spreads to the lungs, to the bone, and to the brain. Then we use other forms of treatment, including radiation therapy, chemotherapy, and hormone therapy in various combinations.

I believe a patient who has advanced or widespread cancer should request a team of specialists, including surgeons, radiotherapists, and chemotherapists; otherwise she may be referred to one type of specialist—say, a radiotherapist—who may treat the malignancy with the method he knows best—in this case, radiation—whether it is the preferable treatment or not. Or she may be referred to a surgeon, who will approach the cancer from a surgical point of view when chemotherapy may be the proper treatment in her case.

How is it decided which treatment to use?

This decision is based on the extent and type of the tumor.

How does radiation therapy work?

In radiation therapy we are firing "bullets" of radiation energy designed to hit the cancerous cells at tremendous speed, thereby causing their destruction. Because sufficient numbers of bullets must be used, radiation therapy can also cause damage to surrounding normal tissue. This problem greatly limits the amount of radiation that can be used, even though normal cells have a greater capacity to recover than cancer cells.

Radiation therapy, combined with chemotherapy, is the best choice only when there is extensive disease and the cancer has spread to the lymph nodes. Under these circumstances, surgery is not effective and may be harmful.

How does chemotherapy work?

Chemotherapy is the treatment of cancer with chemicals. It works by interfering with the ability of the cancer cells to divide or produce certain critical substances necessary for the cells' survival. This, of course, prevents the cancer from spreading, and in certain cancers may actually provide a cure. The beneficial thing about chemotherapy is that it reaches every cell in the body, unlike surgery and radiation therapy, which can only reach specific targets.

Today there are more than forty different drugs used in chemotherapy. Many are used in combination in order to render them more effective.

We hear such horrible things about the side effects of chemotherapy.

There is no question that chemotherapy can make you sick or even cause death. Anytime you deal with strong medicines you are likely to have side effects, and chemotherapy can cause a wide range of problems including damage to the liver, kidneys, and heart. There may be a rapid fall in white blood cells. Less serious side effects are nausea and hair loss. Chemotherapy requires very careful supervision by a physician so that proper doses can be given and the medications can be discontinued if there are any serious problems involving other organs of the body.

Radiation therapy and chemotherapy are both double-edged swords in this regard, but they can be effective in prolonging life and improving the way the patient feels.

What is hormone therapy?

Hormones can be used in the temporary control of some cancers. Testosterone, for instance, the major male hormone, is used in certain breast cancers that are extremely sensitive to female hormones. The use of testosterone is associated with some very disagreeable side effects, such as loss of scalp hair and the development of extensive facial hair. In other types of breast cancer which have no dependence on estrogen, very large doses of this female hormone can be beneficial.

The use of hormones in this way changes the environment of the cancer and reduces its growth potential. Nevertheless, hormone therapy is used less today because of the superiority of chemotherapy.

Is it wise after a mastectomy to have the breast reconstructed by plastic surgery?

This technique is most successful following a simple mastectomy where the breast has been removed because of extensive nonmalignant tumors and cysts, particularly chronic cystic mastitis. Here the lymph nodes are left intact, and a well-trained plastic surgeon can usually perform a breast augmentation without difficulty. To do this he places a silicone implant beneath the skin and nipple of the breast. The cosmetic results are very satisfactory.

The same procedure can often be performed after a modified radical mastectomy for the treatment of cancer, and it's important for women who undergo this surgery to be told that reconstruction is often possible. Here the surgery is much more difficult and expensive since the silicone implant is placed beneath the major muscle under the breast, and a new nipple must be constructed.

In addition to breast cancer, what are the other common female malignancies?

Most often these are cancer of the uterine lining, known as endometrial cancer, and cancer of the mouth of the uterus, known as cervical cancer. Next in frequency comes cancer of the ovaries. Least common are malignancies of the vulva, vagina, and fallopian tubes.

How are these cancers detected?

Different cancers are detected in different ways. Cancer of the cervix can be detected quite early by the Pap test. We have already discussed how important this test is, how accurate, quick, and pain-free. The Pap test will indicate a cancer even when there are no other symptoms. The physician may examine the patient and find nothing wrong, but the Pap test will issue its warning if there is cancer of the cervix, even in the earliest stages. The Pap test, however, is not a reliable detector of endometrial cancer and is useless in detecting ovarian cancer.

Incidentally, a positive Pap smear is not positive proof that cancer exists. A case in point involved a young woman, age twenty-three, who had an abnormal Pap smear and was told that she required a hysterectomy. When the young woman asked for a thorough explanation of her cancer, she was told it was confined to the surface of her cervix (a condition known as carcinoma in situ), but the doctor said he felt it would be best for her to have a hysterectomy. The young woman, who was extremely knowledgeable, had heard there were other approaches to such early cancer, and she asked for a consultation.

When the consultant examined the patient with the colposcope, an instrument which magnifies the cells ten to fifteen times, he felt that the cancer was so very early that he was not absolutely certain it was even cancer at all. The consultant recommended that the suspect cells be frozen by cryosurgery. Although this technique is not always successful, the physician felt he was dealing with a highly intelligent and cooperative patient who would absolutely return for follow-up examinations, so that if the problem did recur it would be detected early. The cryosurgery was performed, and the patient has had perfectly normal Pap tests for the past two years. She has successfully avoided an operation and the loss of her reproductive organs and has had a child. Of course, this type of treatment should only be used by highly qualified gynecologists in carefully selected cases.

How is true cancer of the cervix treated?

If the cancer is just beneath the surface or only half an inch in diameter, it may be treated by radical hysterectomy. This involves removal of half of the vagina, the uterus, the tissue beside the uterus, and the lymph nodes. But one of the ovaries may be saved so that the woman continues to produce estrogen and progesterone. This is particularly important in younger women since the vagina is not damaged by radiation and will return to normal size with use.

If the cancer is more extensive, radiation therapy is the preferable method of treatment.

How is cancer of the endometrium detected?

The most common symptom of endometrial cancer is irregular bleeding with or without abdominal discomfort, both of which must always be reported to the doctor. Sometimes the cancer is uncovered during a routine pelvic examination when the physician feels an enlargement on the uterus. Then he may perform an endometrial biopsy or use one of the various diagnostic washing techniques which suck or wash out the endometrial cells for study. If these cells appear abnormal, a D&C must be performed for a more exact diagnosis. We have already discussed how the D&C involves dilation of the uterus and then a scraping of cells from the uterine wall, which can be studied under the microscope. The biopsy or washing technique should never be used to make a definitive diagnosis of cancer. This can only be done by a D&C.

How is cancer of the endometrium treated?

We generally use radiation first followed by a hysterectomy in a few days or weeks. The radiation step may not be necessary if the cancer is diagnosed very early. Unfortunately the ovaries must also be removed because cancer of the endometrium depends on estrogen to grow.

Are cancers of the cervix and uterus curable?

Approximately 90 percent of those women with small cancers will have at least a five-year survival rate. If the cancer has progressed outside the uterus, however, the chance of survival varies with the extent of the disease and the immune response of the patient. We can never predict the exact outcome of any individual case. A woman with a widespread, seemingly hopeless cancer may have a favorable response to treatment, especially if she places herself in the hands of a competent team and follows their instructions carefully.

I recall one remarkable story about a woman who had cancer of the endometrium and was absolutely convinced that she was going to die. Although her cancer had been detected very early and she had had excellent treatment, she was certain that her cancer was not curable, and she began to prepare herself to die. As a final gesture of love to her family she began knitting three beautiful afghans with very intricate patterns for her children. It took almost three years for her to finish the project, and at that point her physician informed her there was no sign of recurrence of her disease and that in all likelihood she was completely well. Careful examination of her pelvis, bones, and blood revealed that the cancer was gone. With great enthusiasm, the woman presented the afghans to her three children They were so touched they sent both their parents on a trip to South America.

What are the symptoms of cancer of the ovary?

This is the most silent gynecologic cancer and the most difficult to diagnose. Frequently by the time the patient has real symptoms the disease has progressed to the point where treatment is difficult. That is why the survival rate in this cancer has not increased very much in the last five years.

The best advice I can give a woman who has vague abdominal

discomfort, a feeling of persistent indigestion, or pain during sexual intercourse is that she consult her gynecologist and maintain a regular schedule of periodic examinations.

How does the gynecologist make his diagnosis of ovarian cancer?

If the pelvic examination reveals an enlargement of either ovary, the treatment will depend partly on the age of the woman.

If we find a cyst in a teenager or a woman in her early twenties, for instance, we would first place her on oral contraceptives, because these cysts are usually due to the ovulation process, as we have discussed. If, on the other hand, the patient is approaching menopause or is already menopausal, we would perform an immediate exploratory operation. We would open the abdomen, a procedure known as a laparotomy, remove the ovary, and send it to the pathologist for diagnosis. With the patient still under anesthesia we would also examine the entire abdomen. Even then, we cannot always make a definite diagnosis. Some malignancies are questionable, and here the amount of surgery that should be performed is a very critical decision. In women over the age of forty in whom we suspect cancer, the pelvic organs should generally be removed. These women are past their reproductive years. Their ovaries will not function much longer and they are at high risk because cancer of the ovary increases with age.

A more conservative approach is taken with women who are still in their active childbearing years. In these women, we do not remove both ovaries and uterus until a definitive diagnosis can be made, even though this may require two operations.

I might illustrate this problem with a case history of a young woman who came to see me for an abortion. On examining this patient I found a cyst on her right ovary. It seemed to me at that time that the cyst was probably caused by her pregnancy, so I told her to return to the office to be rechecked about four weeks after the abortion. Unfortunately, the cyst was still there four weeks later, so it was important that exploratory surgery be performed.

We opened the patient's abdomen and found a suspicious-looking cyst on her right ovary. I removed the ovary and fallopian tube, but when the pathologist was unable to make a quick diagnosis we closed the patient's abdomen and sent the removed tissue for more complete microscopic studies. But even these results came back questionable. We had a real dilemma, so we explained to the patient that most likely this tumor was of such low-grade malignancy that just removing the ovary would be sufficient to cure her disease. On the other hand, to be completely certain we would have to perform a more extensive operation, although this was something we would prefer not to do in a young woman who has not yet had children.

After explaining the dilemma to the patient, we allowed her to make her own decision. She elected to treat the condition conservatively, that is with removal of the one ovary and tube. It has now been four years without any additional signs of a problem. A decision like this should not be made without the help of a pathologist who has had extensive experience in diagnosing these ovarian lesions.

Of course, if the ovary is definitely diagnosed as cancerous, it is absolutely essential that the uterus, both tubes, and ovaries be removed immediately because cancer of the ovary spreads quickly. This surgery is often followed by chemotherapy. While the prospects for treating cancer of the ovary are not optimistic, the disease may be successfully kept under control for months or even years, particularly if the patient is treated by a team of specialists who work together on her problem. While only a small percentage of patients can be permanently cured, many are able to go on with their lives for long periods of remission with chemotherapy.

A perfect illustration of chemotherapy in action involves a fifty-six-year-old woman who several years ago began to have some enlargement of her abdomen which she first felt was due to weight gain. One afternoon, however, while she was taking a walk she developed a sudden, severe pain in her side. She went to see her physician and a pelvic examination revealed a large ovarian mass. This woman underwent surgery, and she was found to have such extensive cancer throughout her pelvis that it was impossible to remove her reproductive organs. In fact, the cancer had actually spread to her bowel.

One would naturally think this was a hopeless case. Nevertheless, this woman was placed on chemotherapy and after six months her cancer had almost totally disappeared. Now an operation was possible, and the surgeon very correctly reopened this woman's abdomen, performed pelvic surgery, and put the patient back on chemotherapy. It is now eighteen months after this second operation, and this woman leads an entirely normal life without evidence of recurrence of her disease. One doesn't give up with cancer of the ovary, because chemotherapy can be very dramatic and very advantageous.

If a woman has her ovaries removed because of ovarian cancer, is it safe for her to receive estrogen replacement to reduce the severe menopausal symptoms that follow the operation?

This is a source of much misinformation, and there are even some physicians who are not aware that certain ovarian cancers are not dependent on estrogen in order to grow. It is perfectly permissible for a woman to receive estrogen replacement if she has had a hysterectomy and both ovaries removed because of ovarian cancer.

I remember one young woman who came to see me for a checkup when her physician was on a leave of absence. She had had a complete pelvic clean-out because of ovarian cancer, but she had not been receiving estrogen replacement because her physician felt it would be dangerous. The patient had had a particularly difficult time and suffered with severe hot flashes and vaginal changes, to the point where she was unable to have satisfactory intercourse, and she and her husband were finally divorced.

When I checked this woman's record, I found her ovarian cancer was not dependent on estrogen in any way, so I prescribed estrogen pills to be taken orally and estrogen cream for use in her vagina. She immediately began to feel greatly improved. She regained her sex drive and had a very successful, very pleasant affair which restored her self-image. This woman has been totally rehabilitated with the use of estrogen replacement therapy.

Do women who have had a hysterectomy still need routine examinations and Pap smears?

They definitely do, particularly if the hysterectomy was performed because of cancer. There may be some precancerous cells which may later develop biologic changes and become malignant.

Even if the hysterectomy was performed because of some noncancerous disease, such as fibroid tumors, the woman is still able to develop cancer of the vagina, or she may have other abnormalities which must be regularly checked. We call these abnormalities *dysplasia*, and treatment depends on the severity of the problem.

The diagnosis of dysplasia is also made with the aid of a colposcope, which is an instrument that magnifies the cells of the cervix and vagina to detect suspicious areas which should be biopsied. Use of the colposcope is simple, inexpensive, and painless. It is extremely useful in uncovering early changes which may lead to cancer or in determining the extent of various early malignancies of the vagina and cervix.

We haven't discussed cancer of the vulva, or lips of the vagina. How is this disease first detected?

This type of cancer first appears as a lump or sore which the patient and the physician can easily see and feel. Nevertheless, cancer of the vulva has a higher degree of patient and physician neglect than any other type of gynecologic cancer, because patients do not report these lesions, and physicians sometimes prescribe medication without proper examination and biopsy. So if a woman has a lump that does not heal on her vulva, or inside her vagina, she should call it to the attention of her physician. He should perform a biopsy and study the suspicious tissue under the microscope. He should not just prescribe some medication.

How is cancer of the vulva treated?

It is treated surgically by the removal of the vulva, the clitoris, approximately one half of the vagina, and three or four inches of skin on each side of the vulva. Despite this extensive surgery, intercourse is still possible.

I recall a fifty-year-old woman who had this operation. About two and a half months after her operation the patient, who was a warm, very affectionate and loving woman, felt well enough to resume intercourse, but her husband was completely turned off by the appearance of her vulva. Although he tried, there was no way he could make love to his wife, and he refused to allow her to practice fellatio.

The woman felt a deep affection for her husband and tolerated his attitude, but she made no further overtures and presumed their sexual life was over. Then, just by accident, this woman made a business acquaintance with whom she developed a great deal of rapport. They became very close friends and after a period of months he asked her to spend a weekend with him.

At this point, the woman told him quite frankly about her physical condition. The man said he still wanted to spend a weekend with her, so that was arranged, and their lovemaking was extremely satisfactory. This relationship lasted for several years, and during this time the woman remained with her husband, but she continued to have a very satisfactory love affair of which he was unaware.

Is it wise for the woman who has cancer to be treated by her own gynecologist? Or should she be referred to a cancer specialist?

If the cancer has been discovered reasonably early, the woman's own gynecologist can treat her. But if the cancer is moderately advanced, it is preferable that she go to a cancer specialist because she will generally need a team approach.

When I make a diagnosis of cancer, I explain the situation to the patient in simple terms. I say, "Mrs. Jones, the D&C we performed indicates that you do have some malignancy"—I don't usually use the word cancer—"in your womb." Then I go immediately to the positive points, the encouraging points. I may say, "It seems we have found the disease reasonably early, and you have a good chance of a complete cure."

If the cancer is extensive, I would say, "It seems the malignancy has spread beyond the womb, but we are fortunate today that we have a number of things that we can do. We can not only prolong your life, but we can make your life more comfortable and worthwhile, and I am going to refer you to specialists in gynecologic cancer. These specialists, including radiologists, surgeons, chemotherapists, will work together as a team. They have extensive experience with these problems, and they are going to study your case and give you the very best treatment."

What are the most common misconceptions about cancer that you encounter?

The number one misconception is that all women with cancer are going to die from the disease. Another misconception is that women with cancer are unclean and should not have sex. This is the time when these women *need* sex; they require affection and understanding. Intercourse is absolutely safe at this time because cancer is not contagious.

Intercourse is particularly important if the patient has had radiation of her vagina in the treatment of cancer of the cervix or uterus, since coitus will help keep the vagina from shrinking and allow it to maintain its function.

I remember one such young woman with cancer of the cervix who was treated with radiation therapy. In order to prevent shrinkage of the vagina, which radiation will cause, and to break up radiation scar tissue, we asked the patient to have intercourse regularly or at least to regularly insert into the vagina a candle with a condom placed over it. The candle would exert pressure against the vaginal walls in order to maintain the vaginal length and diameter.

This woman's husband was emotionally unable to cooperate either in having intercourse to keep the vagina open or in performing the candle exercises. So the young woman did the candle exercise herself, and eventually went out and found a lover. When her vagina stabilized, she told her husband that she was miraculously improved. She discontinued the love affair, and she and her husband resumed their former sexual relationship.

What other common mistakes are made with regard to cancer?

The very worst thing a woman can do is neglect her treatment. There have been times that we have told patients that they have cancer, and they have ignored our warnings that they must come in for treatment. After a positive Pap test, we have sent registered letters to patients to be sure they have received the results. Nevertheless, some of them have not returned; they have tried to hide from their problems. We have one or two of these cases a year. Sometimes they go to another doctor and don't tell him they had an abnormal Pap test or even that they have been told they have cancer. If he doesn't perform the appropriate tests and make the same diagnosis, they tell themselves they're all right. Needless to say, the results of this sort of wishful thinking are often very tragic.

13
MENOPAUSE

The approach of menopause can be a very scary thing for many women. Some of us view it as the beginning of the end, a downhill path to old age.

Nobody wants to grow old, including me, and this is what makes the menopause so threatening. Women worry about their attractiveness and their physical well-being. But their fears are often based on misconceptions. The truth is that after their body has adjusted to the hormonal changes which do occur, many women are as vigorous as during the years when their bodies were meeting the biological demands of bearing children.

The important thing to remember is that menopause is a normal part of life. Most women have a good chance of coming through with no trouble at all, and the average woman will go on to live another twenty or twenty-five useful years. This is very different from the turn of the century, when life expectancy was around fifty years and the menopause came very near the end of a woman's life.

But so many adjustments have to be made.

This, of course, is the problem. It is during this period that the children leave home; and for the woman who has devoted her entire existence to raising a family, there is suddenly a tremendous void. There is the feeling she is no longer needed as a mother, and she may turn to her husband only to find him preoccupied with business affairs. Marriages are placed under greater stress during this period, and husbands and wives must both go through a time of readjustment.

What is the definition of menopause?

I define menopause as the cessation of menstruation for at least six months. Normal menopause occurs when the ovaries gradually stop producing estrogen.

What causes this to happen?

The aging process causes a slowdown of most body functions, and estrogen production is no exception. Just as many people begin to need bifocals around the age of forty because the lenses of their eyes begin to harden, just as professional athletes begin losing their superb muscular strength and coordination around the age of thirty, the pituitary gland and some of the stimulatory centers of the brain begin to slow down in women around the age of forty. The pituitary begins to produce less and less of its follicle-stimulating hormones which cause the ovaries to function and produce estrogen. There is a gradual cessation of ovulation, and menstruation occurs less and less frequently so that the woman loses her ability to conceive children.

It is easy to see why nature turns off this reproductive process. The woman's arteries are becoming smaller as she ages, and her blood supply to various organs is being reduced. If she were to become pregnant in her late forties or fifties, these pregnancies would be associated with a much higher incidence of hypertension, bleeding problems, labor problems, and birth defects. This is nature's way of preventing these problems. Another reason that a woman stops producing estrogen around the age of fifty is that until this century women seldom lived beyond that age.

At what age does menopause occur?

Usually somewhere between ages forty-eight and fifty-two, but the timing can vary greatly due to health and genetics. Some individuals enter menopause in their thirties, and others do not experience cessation of menstruation until the late fifties. One recent finding indicates that women who smoke are likely to enter menopause at an earlier age.

Can a woman predict when menopause will arrive in her particular instance?

The onset of menopause is determined by several factors—family history, standard of living, race, even the age when a woman began menstruating. It seems peculiar, but the younger a woman was when her periods began, the longer she will continue to have them. If she had the appropriate biologic rhythm to initiate menstruation at the age of ten and a half or eleven, this will generally continue until she is around fifty-five. On the other hand, if a woman began to menstruate at seventeen or eighteen, her menstrual periods will probably cease around the age of forty-five or forty-seven.

The age of onset of menopause is also hereditary. A woman will probably stop menstruating around the same age as her mother and grandmother.

What are the most common symptoms of menopause?

True physical symptoms caused by lowered amounts of estrogen include a reduction in the size of the breasts, vulva, uterus, and vagina, loss of the elasticity of the skin, hot flashes, weakening of the bones (known as osteoporosis), as well as vaginal dryness and itching.

The severity of these symptoms is often a matter of how fast the ovaries stop working. Those fortunate women whose ovaries shut down gradually have an easier time because the hormones from the pituitary which stimulate the ovaries are exhausted slowly, and the adrenal gland has time to take over some of the ovarian responsibility for production of estrogen. In those women whose ovaries stop functioning suddenly because of surgical removal of the ovaries or even because of natural causes, the stimulating hormones remain high, desperately trying to stimulate the inactive ovary to produce estrogen. When the ovary doesn't respond, the hormones try harder and harder, throwing the body's chemistry out of kilter and causing the symptoms mentioned.

How long do menopausal symptoms last?

Menopause is usually a gradual process, and symptoms can last from six months to a number of years, until the body has had a chance to adjust. Many women have no symptoms at all, but for those who do, estrogen replacement therapy is often helpful.

How is estrogen replacement beneficial during the menopause?

I believe that estrogen therapy is helpful in relieving hot flashes, vaginal changes, osteoporosis, and loss of skin tone. In addition, I am told by many postmenopausal patients that estrogen replacement increases their sense of well-being. Since I have no way of measuring the psychological factors involved in their observations, I can only believe them.

I feel that each woman is the world's greatest authority on how she feels. If it is her belief that estrogen enhances her general vigor and approach to life, I am prepared to work with her. I have had postmenopausal patients who began estrogen therapy after several years without hormonal replacement tell me that they resumed erotic dreams after they began estrogen. Who is to say that estrogen did not rekindle their sexual centers?

But isn't estrogen therapy dangerous?

My personal position is that long-term estrogen replacement may be appropriate and beneficial for many patients; and it certainly can be safe when used under a doctor's care as long as the patient undergoes thorough, periodic checkups. After all, nature provides many women with long-term estrogen replacement from their own adrenal gland.

It is important, however, when a woman is about to begin estrogen replacement therapy (ERT) that her physician perform a biopsy of the lining of her uterus. In this way the doctor can tell if there are any abnormalities which should contraindicate the woman's taking estrogen. This procedure should be performed again after the first six months of treatment, and every year thereafter, so the physician can detect changes before they become cancerous. The biopsy, which is a simple office procedure, allows the physician to accurately adjust the dosage of the hormones.

The gynecologist should also take a periodic Pap smear, and perform a periodic breast and rectal examination. Periodic laboratory studies should be performed to check for kidney disease, anemia, and thyroid disorders. If all this is done correctly, the patient will have the lowest risk of cancer that is possible under the present state of our gynecologic surveillance.

Of course, I also believe that patients should be apprised of the present controversy concerning estrogen replacement so they can exercise informed consent concerning therapy. It is extremely important when a woman undergoes any type of therapy or takes any kind of medication that she weigh the benefits she may receive versus the possible risks, and estrogen therapy is no exception to this rule. The fact that the government is now requiring all estrogen prescriptions to be accompanied by an explanatory brochure is a step in the right direction—provided these inserts are carefully prepared and do not offer one-sided information.

It has been my observation that this is not always the case. Some of this information goes into great detail concerning the possible problems which may arise, but it often does not put proper emphasis on the advantages of estrogen therapy in improving the quality of a woman's life by combatting hot flashes, vaginal dryness, and other menopausal symptoms. So giving a woman half-truths is not being helpful. It is distressing to me to think of the number of women in our country who are developing painful intercourse or having unnecessary bone fractures from osteoporosis because they have been frightened away from estrogen therapy by the exaggerated dangers described in package inserts.

What are some possible problems that may arise from estrogen replacement?

Minor side effects may include mild nausea, fluid retention and occasional breast tenderness. Estrogen replacement may also aggravate some previously existing conditions such as migraine headaches, epilepsy, or kidney disease, and it may also cause benign fibroid tumors of the uterus to grow larger. All these problems are quite rare and do not necessarily rule out estrogen replacement. It is those women who have had breast or uterine cancer who should not be given estrogen replacement because these are tumors which are dependent upon estrogen to grow. Women who have had cancer of the cervix or ovary may safely receive estrogen replacement since these cancers are not estrogen-dependent.

I believe it has been incorrectly reported that women using estrogen during menopause may be more likely to develop gall-bladder disease. While this may be the case with women taking estrogen birth control pills, it has not been proven in women taking estrogen replacement during menopause. Neither has it been proven that the use of estrogen during menopause increases the risk of blood clots, but more information is needed for us to be certain.

Women should be informed that the hormones used in menopausal replacement therapy are the same natural and normal hormones which are produced in their own body. These hormones are not to be confused with the hormones in oral contraceptives, which are artificial. The risk factors are in no way comparable.

How should a woman take estrogen replacement?
There are a number of ways in which doctors prescribe estrogen replacement therapy. Estrogen may be taken daily during alternate weeks so there is one week on and one week off the medication. Sometimes the doctor may prescribe that estrogen be taken two or three days of every week. Another schedule is three weeks on and one week off the medication.

Some doctors feel that estrogen should always be taken in conjunction with a progestin. Here the estrogen is used daily for three weeks, then a combination of estrogen and progestin is used for one week. The advantage of this method is that it provides more normal action on the lining of the uterus and is less likely to be associated with cancer of the endometrium.

Can estrogen taken during menopause cause cancer of the uterus?
There are some data to indicate that postmenopausal women taking estrogen for more than one year have a five to ten times greater chance of contracting cancer of the lining of the uterus than women who do not take estrogen. This information, however, is inconclusive be-

cause it was obtained from women who did not have a uterine biopsy before therapy was begun, so there was no way to determine if there was cancer already in existence when the estrogen replacement was initiated. Nor did these women have periodic biopsies while they were taking estrogen replacement. Such biopsies would have detected early abnormalities and enabled the physician to cease therapy before cancer developed. Another problem involved the fact that these women did not receive progestin for three to five days each month along with their estrogen. This progestin would have prevented overgrowth of the lining of their womb. So you see these statistics are not very dependable.

Even though the data are not conclusive, it is possible that the risk of cancer of the endometrium, or lining of the uterus, does increase with the amount of estrogen being taken and with the length of time it is being used. That is why it is important for a woman to take estrogen only under the supervision of a physician who will keep her endometrium and other organs under surveillance.

And one more thing a woman should know about taking estrogen during menopause: any vaginal bleeding should be reported promptly to the physician. While such bleeding may be of no serious consequence, it may be an early warning sign of cancer.

Can estrogen replacement cause breast cancer?

Although this has been found to be the case in laboratory animals placed on high doses of estrogen over relatively long periods of time, there is no way yet to be sure about the effects of long-term estrogen on the human breast. It should be noted, however, that the estrogens that are causing cancers in laboratory animals were given to specially bred animals that had a high natural incidence of breast cancer, and the daily dosages used were several hundred times the daily dose used in humans.

We have heard that estrogen may help prevent heart disease. Is this correct?

There is neither an increase nor a decrease in coronary artery disease with postmenopausal estrogen therapy.

Because the incidence of coronary artery disease begins to rise at just about the time a woman enters menopause, it was originally thought that estrogen replacement might help reduce such disease. Now, well-controlled studies have indicated that estrogen makes no difference.

Interesting data are becoming available, however, concerning smoking. It is now evident that women suffer greater adverse effects from smoking than do men, and are more likely to develop coronary artery disease if they are smokers. So if a woman approaches the age of menopause and is still puffing away, this is even greater reason for her to stop.

How long should a menopausal woman take estrogen? Some physicians say forever, while others say practically never.

If her routine checkups reveal no adverse reactions, I often let the woman herself be the judge of how long she should continue to take estrogen. For several months each year, however, I ask the woman to discontinue her hormones to see how she feels without them.

It has been estimated that over half of all women going through menopause do not require estrogen. Others may need estrogen only long enough to tide them over several months of symptoms while their bodies adjust to lower levels of estrogen.

It is only a small minority of women who require long-term estrogen replacement, but for these women the results can be extremely beneficial.

In addition to taking estrogen, what else can a woman do to keep herself more comfortable during menopause?

There are several drugs that do not contain estrogen that physicians can use to control menopausal symptoms in women who cannot take estrogen. But one thing that is often overlooked is the value of exercise. This can be of tremendous benefit to women who have anxiety, hot flashes, and related problems. The extent of an exercise program should be carefully discussed with the gynecologist, but skipping rope, something most women learn as children, is a very good method. Other good exercises include running in place, easy jogging, tennis, bicycling, and swimming. The type of exercise program used should be discussed with one's physician.

If a woman can afford it, she might enroll in a supervised program of exercise that she can learn and can continue in her own home. Exercise relieves anxiety and tension and is something that I think is of tremendous importance to women who are going through difficult periods in their life.

Which brings up the question, What causes the tension and irritability that many women experience as they approach menopause?

One of the things that disturb me deeply is that women who are nervous and upset around the age of thirty-five or forty tell each other their symptoms are caused by the fact they are entering menopause. This is rarely the case, and these symptoms, in general, are caused by psychological stress and reflect personal factors in the patient's life.

It is also amazing to me how many physicians tell women who have emotional problems during their thirties and forties that their problems are caused by the onset of menopause. This is putting the cart before the horse. Emotional tension is the *cause* of most symptoms, not the result. I feel that some doctors have a tendency to overdiagnose menopause and to place some women on estrogen therapy for emotional problems because that is the easiest thing to do. But there is no way that estrogen can relieve a patient of emotional stress caused by problems in her personal life.

But can't estrogen deficiency be the cause of nervous tension?

While there are occasional patients whose central nervous system is, indeed, affected by lack of hormones, this is relatively rare, and it happens most often in women who have undergone surgical menopause. I remember one young patient who had a total hysterectomy and removal of her ovaries because of severe endometriosis. Right after I performed her operation, I had a severe illness in my own family, and I was called away before I had the opportunity to prescribe estrogen replacement therapy. When I saw this patient about a month later, she described strange periods of depression and crying that she had never had before. She was a well-adjusted woman with a very stable marriage, but her husband also reported that her personality really had changed in the short time since her operation. I immediately placed her on estrogen and progestin and within a week she was entirely back to normal.

So, in answer to your question, yes, estrogen deficiency under certain circumstances can cause nervous tension.

We hear such horror stories about how menopause can cause mental illness.

There are psychological changes in all human beings as they grow older. Men and women alike become more sensitive and possibly more paranoid from the "knocks of life" they have suffered. Thus some women may have an exaggeration of their psychological problems as a result of the added stress of menopause.

I happen to be of the school that menopause, by and large, does not cause emotional problems. It can, however, make existing problems worse. The severe emotional disturbances which occur during menopause are rare, and they usually occur among women who have had previous emotional problems. But even those women who have not had serious emotional difficulties can benefit from short-term psychiatric help at this time.

If women are misinformed about their symptoms, men must be even more so.

Indeed they are! It's too bad that gynecologists don't see their patients' husbands or lovers more often because they also need more accurate information.

The entire family, in fact, may believe the woman's irritability, insomnia, and emotional upheavals are related to menopause and therefore will pass with time. This attitude enables family members to avoid offering assistance to help correct the problems in the woman's life.

But many women find it difficult to talk with their husbands about menopause.

Again, I tell my patients to say that *I* told them to bring it up. Blame it on me. Say, "Dr. Flowers felt I ought to talk to you about this, and here are some of the things he thought you should know: Menopause is a perfectly normal time in a woman's life. Every woman goes through it, and even though I have stopped menstruating, my vagina is perfectly fine. You know, I was afraid I would not be able to make love anymore, but he said I could keep on until I am seventy-five or eighty or even older.

"And you know those hot flashes I have been having? He said they are perfectly normal, and there are things he can do about them. I am going to feel better soon, and indeed, I may feel better than I have in a long time. So I don't want you to worry.

"And another thing. Dr. Flowers said to talk to you about the reasons I have been so nervous and upset lately. He said my nervousness has nothing to do with menopause. He thinks it's because I'm worried about the children moving away. I'm upset because Johnny got arrested for smoking pot, and I'm worried about Mary-Jo going out with that boy I don't like. Dr. Flowers said all these things on my mind are making my symptoms worse, and if I can correct them, I will feel better."

Do many menopausal women bring such personal problems to their gynecologist?

People who have problems carry them everywhere, and if a physician is a good listener, is sympathetic and caring, he can't help but become involved and be helpful.

How do you work with such patients? What exactly do you do?

Sometimes I give them a piece of paper and tell them to list the things that are bothering them most. Then beside each item I tell them to write either, "There is nothing I can do about this," or "There is something I can do about this, and these are my options."

I am trying to get these patients to deal with the difficult situations in their life and to accept what they can't change. It's not often I have to send a patient to a psychologist or psychiatrist.

We women resent being labeled hysterical, aging females who can't cope with our personal lives. Surely some of our menopausal problems are physical in nature.

Some of them are. True hot flashes, vaginal dryness, and even certain minor periods of tension are distinct problems which should be brought to the attention of a physician, who can often help.

Although many menopausal symptoms are, indeed, emotional in nature, many are not, and the physician should perform a thorough evaluation of the patient to be sure. He should take a good history, perform a complete physical examination, and make the necessary laboratory tests. If there is pelvic pain of questionable origin, the physician should look inside the abdomen with a laparoscope so he can be sure about his diagnosis.

What causes the intermittent bleeding that many women experience at the onset of menopause? Is this to be expected?

This is another unfortunate piece of misinformation that women spread among themselves. Menopause is not a license for more frequent bleeding, although such symptoms are common in women in their forties and early fifties. Some of these women bleed for longer periods of time, use more menstrual pads or tampons, and often have bleeding between periods. Although these problems occur frequently, they are never normal—and in 10 to 15 percent of these cases, the irregular bleeding will turn out to be cancerous in origin.

That's why I take the position that all irregular spotting or bleeding which occurs after a woman has ceased her menstrual periods for six months must be considered a sign of cancer until proven otherwise.

The patient with irregular bleeding must always have a thorough examination, a biopsy of her endometrium, and possibly a D&C.

I remember one unfortunate case where a forty-seven-year-old woman neglected irregular bleeding for approximately two years. She thought she was having menopausal changes, and even her physician told her she would "outgrow" it. She was given tranquilizers and injections of hormones at periodic intervals and finally came to see me because she was not improving. Because she had irregular bleeding, I checked first for cancer. I admitted her to the hospital, and a D&C did, indeed, reveal a malignancy. Here was a woman who had had cancer of her uterus for almost two years and who had received inappropriate treatment because she and her physician presumed she was going through menopause.

Of course, not all irregular bleeding is a symptom of cancer. Sometimes the problem is caused by fibroids, polyps or other benign causes. Or there may be a failure of ovulation with a resulting buildup of the lining of the uterus. And often irregular bleeding is caused by a fluctuation of the hormones that control ovulation. We have already discussed how these hormones, which are produced in the brain near the emotional center, are disturbed when a woman is tense and upset. It is for this reason that menstrual irregularity, which so frequently occurs during the onset of menopause, is often a result of psychic and physical fatigue.

Once we have performed an adequate biopsy or a D&C and have established that the irregular bleeding is not caused by cancer or any other physical problem, we must discuss the personal problems in the woman's life so she can correct them or at least deal with them. This often clears up her difficulty with irregular bleeding.

What about the woman who skips menstrual periods?

A woman who misses her menstrual period for several months but then bleeds according to her normal pattern is not menopausal, although she may be approaching the menopausal period of her life. If she is menstruating even three or five times a year, she is producing adequate estrogen and does not require hormone replacement.

Let's talk about the most infamous menopausal symptom of all. What causes hot flashes and debilitating sweats?

Hot flashes occur because of irregularities in estrogen production. Since estrogen has the ability to expand and decrease the diameter of blood vessels, any sudden surge in production of this hormone causes enlargement of the blood vessels near the skin's surface. When the blood rushes in to fill the extra space, the woman feels extremely warm.

Although some women escape hot flashes completely, others have several each day. These annoying episodes may disturb sleep and drench a woman in perspiration—to the point where she must change her night clothes or even her bedding.

It is important for women to realize, however, that not all sweats are menopausal in nature. General anxiety can cause hot flashes all over the body and can also be the cause of night sweats, which can occur at any period in a woman's life. If she is tense and upset her emotional center will be working hard. The emotional factors come to the surface and she wakes up in a cold sweat.

A *true* menopausal hot flash starts above the navel and extends upward, always including the breasts, the neck, *and* the face. When a patient has stopped having menstruation and is having these types of hot flashes, this is definitely a menopausal symptom which can be treated with hormones. We have to make a careful diagnosis, however. If a woman's symptoms are caused by anxiety, we must deal with the problems in her life, because hormones won't help.

Why do the vulva and vagina seem to dry up and atrophy after meno-pause?

The skin in the vagina, as well as the cervix, fallopian tubes, and uterus, is particularly dependent upon estrogen. When the amount of circulating estrogen is reduced, the vagina becomes thin and dry and loses its ability to secrete mucus during sexual intercourse.

The vulva becomes smaller and thinner because of loss of fat, just as loss of fat may occur in the breasts and buttocks. One of the values of estrogen is that it maintains fat in the appropriate areas of the body.

You have mentioned a bone disease called osteoporosis. How is this a menopausal problem?

Osteoporosis is a very common, age-related condition in which the bones of the body become more brittle due to general demineraliza-tion, or loss of calcium. Although the problem occurs gradually, it does not usually produce symptoms until about ten years after the onset of menopause. Patients with osteoporosis frequently develop back pain. Their bones become fragile and have a tendency to frac-ture. They may eventually show other symptoms, including loss of height.

This is one area where we can definitely say that estrogen replace-ment therapy has been proven beneficial.

It is quite possible that more women die from hip fractures related to osteoporosis caused by estrogen deficiency than die from cancer of the uterus which has been estrogen-induced.

Is it wise for a woman to use tranquilizers, antidepressants, and sleeping pills to help her through a rough period?

I find these medications useful on a temporary basis as long as a woman uses them correctly and understands they are being prescribed as a crutch to help her over some difficult periods in her life, much as she would use a crutch or walking stick when she sprains her ankle. She must realize, however, that she is not "naturally nervous" or "naturally depressed." There are complexities in her life that are causing these feelings, and the sooner she deals with them the sooner she can throw the crutch away and avoid dependence on tranquilizers, which can be quite addictive.

What happens to a woman's body after menopausal symptoms subside?

By this time the menstrual periods will have ceased and the ovaries will have gradually stopped all estrogen production. After a certain period of time, which varies among individuals, the hormones which govern reproduction (the follicle-stimulating and luteinizing hormones) also disappear.

Then, in a process known as "peripheral conversion," the adrenal gland begins to take up the slack by producing an estrogen known as estrone sulfate. Surprisingly this estrone is made from an androgen, or male hormone, produced in the woman's body. Those women whose adrenal gland does an adequate job of producing this estrogen will exhibit fewer signs of aging. Unfortunately not all women have this capacity, and they are the ones who will benefit from long-term estrogen therapy.

Many women find it difficult to control their weight after menopause. Is there a physical reason for this?

Although most weight gain is caused by exercising too little and eating too much—often from sheer boredom—there may be additional factors involved in weight gain during menopause. I have a theory that just as nature increased a pregnant woman's capacity to store fat so that she and her baby would not be undernourished should a food shortage occur in primitive societies, it is quite possible that nature gave this same ability to older men and women because they, too, would be unable to go out and hunt their own food supply. This tendency for weight gain during middle age may have been built in for survival's sake during the earlier stages of human development.

Some of us worry that our sex lives may change after menopause. Will we still be able to feel passion?

If a woman was having great sex before menopause, she should continue to have great sex after menopause. Whether she has a functioning uterus or ovaries has very little to do with passion. In fact, many women actually experience an increase in their sexual enjoyment after menopause because they are free from their fears of pregnancy. As the French have long noted, there must be a bit of gray in a woman's hair before she can be a really great lover.

It must be remembered, however, that sex depends largely on one's state of mind. So if a woman is greatly concerned about her aging, feels sorry for herself and is depressed, she is going to have a reduction in her sexuality. On the other hand, if she is vigorous, exercises, and has an inquiring mind, she should continue to have a good sex life. Although it is true that her partner's desire for intercourse will begin to decline with age and she herself may have to use some vaginal lubrication to combat dryness or shrinkage of the vagina, there is no reason that a woman cannot continue to enjoy sex and be orgasmic into her seventies and eighties.

When I was in the Middle East several years ago, I was surprised when several men who were out hunting with me asked if a woman after the age of fifty could have sex. Men in Iran, the Middle East, and even some Western cultures believe that the act of coitus is designed merely to satisfy a man. Because women in these cultures have been treated solely as sexual objects, they use menopause as an excuse not to have sex anymore.

Even in our country, many men mistakenly believe a woman is old after menopause. When a husband finds out that his wife is not menstruating, he may begin to think, "Maybe I shouldn't make love to her anymore. Maybe she won't be able to make love or maybe I am going to hurt her. Maybe I won't be able to bring her to the same sexual heights as before." He may even tell himself, "Now I have a good excuse to have a mistress."

I'd like to tell you a story about a sixty-year-old woman who came to see me recently. Her husband had been dead for about four years, and when I asked if she was having intercourse, a big smile came over her face. "Dr. Flowers," she said, "I had not had intercourse until last week, but it was absolutely wonderful. I reached an orgasm just like I did many years ago, and I felt terrific about this. The man had been just a casual acquaintance, but I thanked him for showing me I could function so superbly."

I think this is a great love story. Here was a woman who had worried that her sexuality was going to be covered by the snow, and that there would never be another spring. Suddenly she discovered that her sexuality was still present and it could be brought out with appropriate stimulation.

Which raises the question, How long should a menopausal woman use contraception?

If a woman forty-five years or older has had no menstrual period whatsoever for six consecutive months, she is probably no longer able to become pregnant. But if she is still having any periods at all, even though they may be infrequent, she is probably still able to conceive. Many women in their late forties do, in fact, become pregnant because they are not diligent about using contraception. This can raise all sorts of medical problems, and middle-aged pregnancies often result in abnormal babies. That's why it is important for a pregnant woman over the age of thirty-five to have the procedure known as amniocentesis, which we discussed when we talked about pregnancy. Amniocentesis may be able to help determine the state of the baby's health.

What if a menopausal woman is frustrated sexually because she has lost her husband or because her partner has lost interest in sex?

If a woman doesn't have a sexual partner, she will gradually lose her desire unless she maintains her own sexuality in some fashion.

If she doesn't want to acquire a lover, I encourage her to masturbate at periodic intervals, maybe two or three times a month. I advise her to set the stage properly, to put on a pretty nightgown, to turn on some nice music, and as she masturbates to fantasize about the different men she may have known, such as former lovers or her deceased husband. Or she may prefer to fantasize about people she would like to have known, movie stars, etc., as the case may be. I also feel there is every good reason for her to use a vibrator around her clitoris in order for her to become orgasmic.

I feel strongly that if a woman does not maintain her sexual interest in some way, if she puts her sexuality in the deep freeze, she may lose her interest forever. And if two or three years later she becomes interested in another lover, she may have great difficulty rejuvenating her sexual desire.

But many middle-aged women have hang-ups about masturbation.

I had one such patient just recently. She is a fifty-seven-year-old college professor who lost her husband several years ago. This woman needed hormone replacement, and during our conversation I discussed the matter of masturbation. Although she had enjoyed a very good sex life with her husband, she felt that masturbation was something she could not do—even though she was able to laugh at the old stories that masturbation would make hair grow on the palms of her hands, make her go crazy, or cause her to become cross-eyed. She did, however, take my advice and tried to fantasize about sex.

Recently this woman came back for a six-month checkup and told me that she had met a man whom she found very attractive. They had intercourse, and she was pleased to find she could still be orgasmic. As a matter of fact, she was actually euphoric over it, and she felt that her continuing feelings of sexuality were a tremendous help in her adjustment to the aging process.

As our bodies begin to show signs of aging, some of us feel we are no longer sexually attractive.

If a woman thinks of herself as a sexual being, if she recognizes and nourishes her own sexual feelings as she grows older, she will continue to be sexually attractive, despite the fact that she is aging. It is true that she may develop lines in her face and her breasts may not be firm, but if she maintains a warmth of sexuality, if she develops a maturity of expression of that sexuality which is associated with understanding, thoughtfulness, and tenderness, she can be far more sexual than a young girl who is merely expressing a biological reflex and urge.

How do you feel about plastic surgery during menopause to bolster a woman's ego?

I have known a number of women who have received a great emotional lift from plastic surgery of the face and breasts. And I am enthusiastic about doing vaginal repairs if a woman feels her vagina is too flabby and large.

I remember one particularly delightful widow of considerable financial means who had decided to marry again. She came in to discuss several matters. First she mentioned that she would like a breast uplift because her breasts were a bit flabby. Then she said she would also like a facelift, and finally she admitted that she felt her vagina was too big. Her late husband had complained about this problem, and she wanted a plastic repair on the vagina so it would be more like that of a younger woman.

It seemed to me that all these things were very reasonable, and we arranged for a plastic surgeon. He did a superb job of putting in breast implants so she had very beautiful breasts. He also took out the crow's-feet around her eyes, and she certainly looked seven or eight years younger. Finally, because the patient had previously had a hysterectomy, it was simple to reduce the size of the vagina and improve its general ability for muscular contractions. The patient was extremely pleased, later remarried, and now tells me how she tries to talk other women into the same approach.

So anything a woman can do to improve her self-image can be of tremendous benefit. That's why I think it is foolish for a patient not to utilize those services available in modern medicine, be it plastic surgery, estrogen therapy, or whatever.

INDEX